P9-DEB-961

MATERNITY
WARD

MATERNITY WARD

Behind the Scenes
at a Big City Hospital

Susan Stanley

WILLIAM MORROW AND COMPANY, INC.
NEW YORK

For Jessie and Katy,
my wonderful daughters

Printed in the United States of America

1-55710-022-5

PREFACE

When I began working on *Maternity Ward*, the plan was to take a close look at, and describe, the inner workings of a large city hospital's labor and delivery department. Because I live in the city of Portland, Oregon, its area citizenry exceeding a million, and because I knew it would be a long haul, I chose to set my book in an already familiar venue.

Working as a free-lance journalist in Portland, I had written a number of times about "Pill Hill," as Oregon Health Sciences University is known, sometimes affectionately, sometimes not. For purposes of my book, there was the added appeal of the university's fertility clinic, its management of high-risk pregnancies and deliveries, and the well-known care given to Multnomah County's welfare recipients and other indigent patients. I would set down the stories of the people who work there—the staff doctors and nurses, the ancillary workers, the medical and nursing students, the residents in Pill Hill's four-year OB/GYN program.

The majority of women delivering at OHSU are indigent—either "welfare" patients surviving on regular public assistance, or simply members of that rapidly expanding class in America whose employment provides no medical benefits and who can ill afford medical insurance on their own. A significant number of middle-class women, however, also make their way up to The Hill.

In my own time on 4NE, Pill Hill's Labor and Delivery Department, I knew I would meet staff doctors, men and women teaching and overseeing the work of increasingly experienced residents, helping them progress from managing ordinary vaginal deliveries toward often complicated cesarean sections—slicing open the bellies of women to bring forth their babies. I would get to know the residents, the young men and women who, after four years of college and another four years of medical school, were now on the last, exhausting leg of their journeys toward qualification in their specialty. Their four-year residencies are served on a grueling schedule, with one hundred-hour work weeks not uncommon. Neglecting their families, often ignoring their own physical and mental health, fueled by adrenaline, frequent infusions of caffeine, sugar—and idealism—they make potentially life-and-death decisions about women and their babies as a matter of routine.

With two daughters of my own, born more than two decades earlier, I imagined that once the dust had settled, once I had grasped new concepts and language, I would find myself on comfortably familiar ground.

I could not have been more mistaken, or more naïve.

For three weeks, I spent every three-to-eleven P.M. evening shift on 4NE. I dressed in baggy green scrubs, the two-piece, V-necked, tied-waist uniform worn by all who work there—housekeeping crew, medical and nursing students, nurses, midwives, and doctors, including the residents and department chairman. Reporter's pad in hand, minicassette recorder tactfully tucked into the breast pocket of my scrubs, I drifted in and out of labor and delivery rooms. Though I clearly identified myself as a nonstaff member, my scrubs-suited presence blended in quickly, becoming part of the maternity ward hubbub. Wearing mask, paper hair snood, and booties, I recorded the details of cesarean sections performed in the two operating rooms. Chronicling all that transpired in a series of single evenings was impossible: Reporters are no more omnipresent than doctors are omniscient.

I talked closely with dozens of the women who come to The Hill to deliver their infants, talked as well with their families. I met their other children, some of whom were in the room when their siblings came mewling and screaming into the world. I spoke with their husbands and boyfriends, watched the birthing women's own parents transformed into ancestors.

Doctors and nurses, students and staff, patients and, by default, newborn humans willingly shared their stories. Sitting in the coffee/supply room, gulping down more than my own share of caffeine and refined sugar, sometimes holding the hand of a laboring woman, I listened to the lives of these people. A charming and cheerful resident's firstborn, I discovered, had been lost to Sudden Infant Death Syndrome. A staff doctor once faced a heartrending ethical choice when his wife was pregnant with twins, one healthy, the other almost surely doomed. Some of them agonizing over their own apparent infertility, nurses and residents worked intimately and uncomplainingly, night after night after night, with laboring women.

Each month, 200 to 250 babies are born on 4NE. But that statistic hardly tells the story; it certainly doesn't reflect the enormous degree of constant, grinding stress. Close to half of those two hundred-plus deliveries qualify as "high risk"—teenage mothers, or women over thirty-five; women whose fetuses suffer from intrauterine growth retardation; women who are bleeding, or have high blood pressure; those who have been using damaging drugs while pregnant. As a center for high-risk pregnancies, much of the work in this labor and delivery department is to *prevent* labor, to keep these women from delivering too early. The objective then, as now, was "a good outcome" for mother and child.

All that is known about both mother and child may be what is on the chart, if there *is* a chart. The patient may be a prostitute, the wife of another doctor on Pill Hill—or a doctor herself. No matter. Residents and nurses are thrown together with a woman for what may well be the most important, intense, dramatic day of her life. And then the child is born, and rerouted elsewhere: to the Mother-Baby Unit, or to the intermediate care nursery, or to the children's hospital in another part of the rat's maze of elderly buildings. Or even, on sad occasion, down to the basement morgue.

The high-tech facilities and procedures of a modern American hospital are mind-boggling. Ultrasound scans of *in utero* infants are routine, and laboring women are, as an immediate matter of course, hitched up to fetal heart-monitoring equipment. (Some critics find all this unnecessarily intrusive; surely the malpractice suits seeking legal revenge for the less-than-perfect baby have produced an understandable terror on the part of the OB/GYN community.)

But what makes today's maternity ward most different from that of the 1960s, when I bore my daughters, is our culture's widespread use of drugs. Licit and illicit drug use by pregnant women has drastically changed how women and their babies, born and unborn, are treated. A laboring woman being admitted to the hospital is routinely queried about her use of drugs, "recreational" or otherwise.

Like any institution, a hospital reflects the society it serves. Unlike most other institutions, however, a hospital offers a clear and unobstructed view of the traumas a society is going through. Downstairs, The War On Drugs routes its wounded straight to Pill Hill's Emergency Room, populating it with the bullet-riddled, knifed bodies of young members of the Bloods and the Crips, L.A.-based, drug-fixated gangs (not that drug-related violence is limited to the young). Upstairs in 4NE, the victims of America's War On Drugs are even younger.

Obstetrics in late-twentieth-century America is being practiced—waged—smack in the middle of a war zone. Very conservatively put, one in ten babies born in American hospitals is, in medical parlance, "drug exposed." Mostly, and very dangerously, these babies are born addicted to crack, the smokable, affordable-to-all form of cocaine. In the Labor and Delivery Department of Oregon Health Sciences University, the doctors and nurses scoff at this statistic. One in five, they say. That's more like it.

I could have chosen instead to don scrubs and haunt the labor and delivery rooms of one of the bottom-line institutions, those full-service private hospitals offering "birthing suites," yoga classes, makeup consultations, and elaborate weight-loss regimens to shed those twenty extra postpartum pounds. In

8

such hospitals, I am told, patient drug use is present; it is simply not discussed.

From the start, I knew my choice of hospital would result in stories that are distressing and raw, perhaps upsetting to some readers. Yet I believed (and still believe) it important that *Maternity Ward* describe a hospital serving all kinds of families, from all walks of life. Descriptions about the work lives of 4NE's staff are literal, and the nurses, doctors, residents, and medical and nursing students appear here as accurately as I could present them. Their real names are used. To protect their privacy, I have chosen pseudonyms for patients and their families, adjusting particulars about occupations, physical appearance, and where they live. Details about their deliveries, and of their medical conditions, however, are accurate and literal.

Susan Stanley
Portland, Oregon

CONTENTS

CHAPTER ONE

DAY 1: Monday, April 11

("She smokes crack, but she's never shot up," says the boyfriend.)

WHEE-OO! WHEE-OO! WHEE-OO! To those working in 4NE, the siren is white noise—unheard, unnoticed, a single thread woven into the audio fabric wrapping the work lives of the dozen or so nurses, residents, students, and other staff. As for the patients, grunting and groaning, panting and relaxing between labor pains, the slowly ticking clock on the wall makes more noise than any siren could.

Outside on this sunny April afternoon, an ambulance is arriving at the Emergency Department four floors down. But things are quiet up on the hospital's northeast wing, the fourth-floor Labor and Delivery Department at Oregon Health Sciences University. The clock on the wall behind the nurses' station reads 3:15, 1515 in medspeak. Behind the nurses' station, in the small room serving as supply center and coffee room, Evening Charge Nurse Denise Reed is informing the four other evening shift nurses of a new policy.

You can't make reference to the HIV test, or its results, in talking with or about a patient, she tells them. But you can say she has AIDS. Get it? Drinking their coffee, the women smile and shake their heads over the logical inconsistency.

Suddenly, Unit Secretary Diane Kuriatnyk pokes her curly head around the corner to tell them about the call just in from the ER.

A team is on its way in with a street woman and her baby just born in the ambulance with the unnoticed siren. Get ready.

Within seconds of this announcement, the elevator door at the end of the hall jerks open. Two ambulance attendants run down the long corridor, pushing a trolley with the woman and her baby riding on top. A skinny young man trots alongside, his face contorted as he awkwardly pats his girlfriend's thin arm. After a noisy, hurried conference in front of the nurses' station, the trolley is shoved into OR1, the operating room on the left. Outside OR1, there in the hall, the ambulance attendant tells of how he delivered the baby: "It wasn't very thrilling," he says. "It was, 'Oh, *sheesh!*'" Nobody is listening to him.

Inside OR1, First-Year Resident Tracey Delaplain—pregnant, tired, up for far too many hours to take all this in stride—delivers Cammie Edwards's placenta. No need to repair any tear on the perineum. In the hall outside the operating room, her jumpy, skinny boyfriend loudly announces to everybody, to nobody in particular, that she's been living on the streets, y' know, and he's just caught up with her, see? Yeah, so she's got a history of drug abuse, and so she smoked crack last night. So? But she's never shot up, *no way,* man!

As he babbles on, his tiny son is—swiftly, silently—bundled up and taken down the hall, carried by a nurse wearing green scrubs, straight into the INCU, the Intermediate Neonatal Care Unit. Here he will begin his long withdrawal from crack cocaine. And from whatever else his mother has been sharing with him.

In a half hour or so, Cammie Edwards, the young mother, is transported by gurney downstairs to the Mother-Baby Unit on 3NW. She's twenty, but looks fourteen, with a delicate dusting of freckles, bright red hair, and that almost transparent skin redheads often have. Though thin, very thin, she is lovely. She is also still so stoned that she hasn't quite got it: that she has just been delivered of her third child, the tiny red-haired son she will call Timothy.

In the INCU down the hall, baby Timothy would have

problems enough being born two months ahead of term, agree the nurses, who've seen it all before. This time, at least, they know which drug the baby's mother has been using—one of them, anyway. They dry the baby off, stimulate him to see if he'll cry. Right now, he's limp as a rag doll, wanting only to sleep. But this will change, the nurses know, even as they diaper him and wrap him snugly in warmed cotton flannel blankets printed with bright baby animals. Placed into a small bed, he'll be hooked up to the heart monitor with the display screen above.

If Timothy Edwards is true to form—and the nurses know he will be—within a few hours of departing his mother's womb, the tiny drug addict will begin to shudder convulsively through a violent withdrawal. There will be high squeaking noises instead of crying. His face will be a miniature study in confusion, fear, and anxiety. He won't be able to get the hang of sucking, so he can't be fed by bottle for the first couple of days.

The nurses in the INCU will "chart" it all. And downstairs in the Mother-Baby Unit, Cindy Shepard and the other nurses looking after Timothy's mother will chart all that they will see in the next few days. The baby's father is cramming Hostess Twinkies into his mouth as he bounces around, trying to talk to anyone who comes into his girlfriend's room. If she follows form—and the nurses know damned well she will—Cammie Edwards will sleep off her drugs, then be completely apathetic until her boyfriend returns, bearing gifts of an evidently psychotropic nature. Whereupon she will become, briefly, very animated.

Through it all, when her baby is brought to her, she'll stare at him. Smiling, smiling, like he's . . . oh, say, a bowlful of potato salad. Or a doll viewed through the toyshop window in a dream she had once, long ago.

They call him "DDH." That's for Darling Doctor Hoffman. Right now, First-Year Resident Gary Hoffman has been on duty for . . . what is it now? Thirty hours, thirty-five maybe? Awake for one hell of a lot longer than that. Awake for two days, bloodshot eyes and all, Gary Hoffman looks like a cross between Tom Selleck and the young Cary Grant. The thick dark brown hair and the lustrous moustache don't hurt the effect any. And then there's that deep cleft in the chin. The consensus among his colleagues of both genders is that men this good-looking don't often come this nice. In fact, Dr. Amanda Clark wishes she had a dollar for every female who, seeing DDH for the first time, stopped dead in her tracks and began making immediate, slack-jawed rearrangements in her own life. To a woman, invariably, they ask it: "Who *is* that? Is he *married?*" Even after they hear the rumor that he tends to vote a straight Republican ticket.

Patients go for DDH in a big way, too. Downstairs in the Mother-Baby Unit, in fact, Debbie Pellegrini, brain-damaged, palsied, in her twenties, knocked up by God-knows-who, is in the habit of grabbing spasmodically toward his crotch whenever Dr. Gary Hoffman drops by to check up on her.

Down the hall in Special Delivery, between contractions LaTonya Jordan keeps telling her mother to make that cute doctor come back in. LaTonya is thirteen and black, and at this moment she hurts all over. Her belly looks like there's a soccer ball inside and she's scared to death at the idea of something that big forcing itself out from between her legs. Her breasts are enormous, more huge than ever with the pregnancy. Their size contrasts strangely with her hair, two dozen or so tiny braids secured with little bright-hued plastic barrettes. A "flesh-colored" Band-Aid dangles in sharp relief against the darkness of her left heel.

With each contraction, LaTonya is crying—*Wah! Wah! Wah!*—keeping her eye on the television screen above, where cartoon creatures called Smurfs frolic in plotless delight. Her mother, a tall-thin-and-elegant-looking woman of perhaps twenty-eight years, her skin a lustrous gleam of pale amber, snaps her fingers and writhes in time to what's coming into her head from her Walkman. (And from whatever it is she's whacked out on this sunny spring afternoon.) Every now and then, she boogies over to her weeping daughter and laughs mirthlessly.

"I *told* you so," she says in a singsong voice, surprisingly mellifluous. "I *told* you what it was gonna be like!"

Down on the second floor, around the corner from the OB/GYN outpatient clinic, Dr. E. Paul Kirk sits behind his desk, his mouth a grim line as he goes over the department's monthly budget figures. A tall, imposing Englishman with a wry, often unexpected sense of humor, the forty-nine-year-old has told his assistant, Susan Mootry, to hold all calls and just take messages while he spends an essential and unusual hour alone in his second-floor office with its soft gray walls and tweedy gray carpet.

At least a dozen large trees, maybe two, died to produce the quantity of paper that, in one form or another, dwells in the office of Dr. E. Paul Kirk, chairman of the Department of Obstetrics and Gynecology of Oregon Health Sciences University. To the left of the doorway are floor-to-ceiling bookcases, a few pictures of his four children placed among the thick and somber tomes dealing with the practice of obstetrics and gynecology. Thirteen black-framed diplomas and certificates fill the wall to Dr. Kirk's right, its window alcove holding a vase filled with pussy willows. The department chairman's desk is placed at a right angle to the wall, presenting no barrier of "authority" between chairman and visiting staffers, students, or residents. To his right, next to the desk, is a four-drawer filing cabinet. An extension off the side of the desk is piled with still more stacks of files.

Against the wall on the other side of his desk is a light-colored wood cabinet, some six feet long, sliding doors below, its top crowded with bulging folders and a paper-crammed brown accordion file. In front of him, on the walnut desk with black melamine surface, are precariously stacked files straining in their folders. Dr. Kirk's desk also holds a small tape recorder for dictation, a vertical metal file holder, two piles of books about obstetrics and gynecology, a telephone in that lurid avocado-green hue refrigerators used to come in, and a mug of strong tea.

His silver-plated Cross fountain pen poised over a sheet of figures, Dr. Kirk takes an automatic sip of the cold tea, then grimaces. Rising from his imitation-leather swivel chair, he takes the few steps across the carpet to a small table in front of the bookcases. There, he switches on an electric tea kettle, drops a Murchie's tea bag into a clean mug, and returns to his desk. The constant buzz of the green phone is answered somewhere else.

By juggling, by making hard choices—again, again, again—it all works out. But the department chairman feels the usual crush, and the usual despair, over the continuing, possibly permanent, dilemma. Namely, it makes no sense, none whatsoever, to have appealing outpatient facilities and lousy inpatient space. The OB/GYN clinic, on the second floor of the hospital's outpatient facilities, is fine. The waiting area is carpeted, with nice upholstered sofas and chairs. Though small, the examination rooms are well equipped, bright and cheerful. It could be a women's clinic anywhere. Not a hint of its predominantly welfare and indigent clientele.

Up in 4NE, the Labor and Delivery Department is another matter indeed. Put plainly, the best that can be said is that L&D looks like some turn-of-the-century charity hospital. "Spare" would be about the kindest description. The five delivery rooms, with the exception of the room called "Special Delivery," are entirely too small, scarcely accommodating the delivery bed and a chair or two for the family and friends who so often nowadays are part of the show. Tuck a couple of residents, a nurse or two, a medical student, and perhaps a student nurse into one of those rooms, and it's a mob scene—untidy, confusing, and very possibly unsafe.

All too often, the PAR—the postanesthesia recovery room—and the prep room down the hall are redefined as delivery rooms. Sometimes, normal vaginal deliveries take place in one of the two operating rooms, simply because the other rooms are filled. (For that matter, in a pinch, the hallway has had to serve, a screen dragged over for a modicum of privacy, if there's time.) There have been efforts, God knows, to improve L&D's physical setup. Some of the nurses, in fact, even came in on their off-hours and painted and papered a couple of the delivery rooms. There are framed posters and prints in the halls and most of the rooms. But the university administration, eyes firmly fixed upon the bottom line, can't expect Pill Hill's L&D to attract the paying customer. Most of the women who come here to have their babies do so because they have little choice. Poor, and either on welfare or uninsured—lacking health coverage of any sort—they drive up the winding road to The Hill, knowing that they will be taken in, that they can have their babies here. They won't be turned away.

But in this day of medicine as big business—and a vigorously competitive one at that—the university constantly pushes Dr. Kirk to attract those private, paying patients. The ones with heavy-duty medical insurance to pungle up for their deliveries. Granted, a number of those private, paying patients come to The Hill for their prenatal care, don't mind rubbing shoulders with the poorer women in the setting of the department's perfectly adequate, attractive outpatient clinic. But actually give birth upstairs in 4NE? In a tiny, nondescript room, with hardly enough room for you and the staff, much less your family? (And never mind about the food!) No way. They want to go to St. Vincent's out on Southwest Barnes Road, or to Good Samaritan on Northwest Twenty-third Avenue, or to North Portland's Emanuel. For their bucks, they want the trimmings.

And who can blame them? A woman remembers the details of her labor all her life, and she wants the birthing experience to be terrific. She wants tasteful, luxurious decor, a stereo in the room, with a big squishy armchair for her husband to sit in. And when all is said and done, once her baby has arrived, she wants a nice dinner with a decent wine, not *hospital food,* to be able to receive her enraptured family and friends in a room with nice carpet and draperies, and nicely papered walls. To be treated like a queen after what is, after all, one of the most important, wonderful moments of her life. The other hospitals know this, and they cater to it: Each month, households throughout the tricounty area receive glossy brochures touting the birthing facilities of this hospital or that. *Have your baby here! We have the newest, shiniest, most personal setting for your glorious experience!*

Dr. Kirk is trying to deal with this latter-day consumer mentality of the paying maternity patient, attempting to reconcile the needs of these finer folk with those of the high-risk patients, with those of the dozens of crack-addicted patients and their damaged, premature newborns. He is trying to come up with some realistic approach to the young women who breeze in, advanced in labor, stoned into some dreamy hinterland. At present, in the city of Portland, Oregon, there is not one program for pregnant women addicted to drugs.

It all comes down to money. Who has it, and who doesn't.

Who "deserves" to have it spent on her care, and on the care of her baby, before and after its emergence into the world.

Even though the American and British medical systems practice equivalent medicine, and speak roughly the same language, the two systems are vastly different in a number of ways. The National Health Service, Britain's scheme of socialized medicine, assures medical care to all of Her Majesty's subjects. For his part, Dr. Kirk went from family practice through a second grueling regimen of training as an obstetrician/gynecologist. Finishing up the second round of training for this specialty in the mid-1970s, he came to question his place in British medicine.

The flavor of union intervention in all levels of daily life in England had become intolerable. Sick people, in his view, were held hostage by striking laundry workers who caused hospital operating rooms to close for lack of sanitary supplies. Private medical practice would apparently soon be phased out for Health Service doctors, many of whom found it necessary to have such a practice in order to support their families. Dr. Kirk's chance meeting with an American doctor led to a job-seeking tour of the United States. He was hired as coordinator of the residency programs at three Portland hospitals: Emanuel, Good Samaritan, and Oregon Health Sciences University.

Appropriately, the Kirk family arrived in Portland on Labor Day, 1975. Dr. Kirk counts himself lucky to have squeaked in under the wire. In 1976, deciding there were too many doctors in the United States, the U.S. government began severely restricting their entry into the country. Nowadays, it's almost impossible for a foreign-born medical graduate to enter the States—not without a long, long wait. And then, once here, long-completed training often must be repeated. British training is still not accepted over here.

For the first two or three years, Dr. Kirk spent one third of his time at each of the three hospitals: Emanuel, Good Samaritan, and OHSU. Other positions followed, including his appointment as assistant chairman of Pill Hill's OB/GYN Department. When the chairman, Leon Speroff, left the school, the Englishman became acting chairman, and then—to his own surprise—was appointed chairman.

It is, at the very least, an unusual appointment, given that he has no national reputation. National contacts, yes, but no vast body of publications or nationally held offices. His credentials as an academician are based on his interest in teaching, and on his providing a role model in the clinic setting, working directly with patients.

Dr. Kirk is highly respected among his colleagues, even the overworked, often cranky residents. He has worked to help establish a midwifery practice at the hospital, and the nurses and residents work alongside the midwives. His sensitivity toward patients is well known. Under Dr. Kirk's aegis, a protocol has developed for the compassionate handling of fetal demise, helping bereaved parents deal with the stillborn and early deaths that, alas, happen from time to time. When the occasional resident is ill—or even, as sometimes occurs, jumps ship midresidency—he has been known to arrange for staff doctors, including himself, to pitch in, spreading thinner the extra work created by the defection. And he "takes call," serving as the staff doctor overseeing the residents, as often as—or more than—other staffers.

And while the Englishman struggles with deficient inpatient facilities, the hospital and university administrators, in turn, struggle with administrators like Dr. Kirk. It is frustrating, dealing with this department chairman, this man who argues with such fierce and reasoned calm that the hospital's responsibility is to look after the patients who have only one choice for their health care. Who believes that it's both appropriate and necessary to target as desirable patients these welfare mothers and their children, to care for the working poor whose scant incomes do not allow for extras. Like health insurance for themselves and their children.

Dr. Kirk thoroughly grasps the dilemma the university faces as it struggles with the Oregon legislature, which keeps repeating that the state is not going to subsidize the institution, that it is high time the hospital and the university paid their own way. And always, Dr. Kirk and the hospital administrators struggle together with the competitiveness that exists in corporate medicine, battling together an overwhelming interest in bottom-line profit, an interest that Dr. E. Paul Kirk views as superseding a concern for the most important question: What is the best health system for the community?

There are a couple of ways to get up to Oregon Health Sciences University's fourth-floor Labor and Delivery Department. After driving up the steep, winding roads of Marquam Hill to the area dubbed "Pill Hill," with its rat's maze of buildings connected by walkways and elevators, you can walk into one of several entrances to North Hospital.

From South Hospital, you can walk over. Or, as many a pregnant woman does, you can waddle over, supported by the strong hands of mother, father, boyfriend, husband, woman friend, or, as is often the case, a combination thereof. Then, making your way through hallways that twist one way then another (asking directions of anyone who looks less confused than you), you come to the far end of North Hospital. Then a flight of stairs, or the elevator, will take you to the fourth floor, called 4NE.

Or you can park your car in the lot surrounded on two sides by North Hospital, and on a third by Emma Jones Hall, where student nurses once dwelt in chaste and chaperoned purity in the century's early years. Entering that far end of North Hospital, you can take either of two dingy, musty-smelling elevators to the fourth floor.

Beyond the double doors, portals to Labor and Delivery, lie the five official labor and delivery rooms, and the PAR and prep rooms that sometimes pinch-hit for L&D, the two operating rooms, and the supply areas. Across the hall from the L&D rooms lies the Intermediate Neonatal Care Unit, a halfway house of sorts for the "feeders and growers," the premature babies who can't suck well yet, and need to put on weight, and sometimes have *apnea*, forgetting to breathe while sleeping. Or the ones whose mothers are probably not going to take them home—by choice or otherwise.

1750: 5:50 P.M.

Staff Perinatalogist Dr. John Bissonnette is leading Board Rounds. Gathered around the nurses' station on this Monday afternoon are three nurses, two medical students, a nursing student, and a pregnant First-Year Resident who swears she will not, repeat *not,* have her baby here when the time comes. They are looking at The Board, on the wall behind the high counter curving above the desk area. The nurses' station is L&D Central, an island of stability amid an ever-shifting sea of activity.

On The Board are listed the facts about each patient currently occupying a labor and delivery room. Her name and age. Where she's been receiving her prenatal care, if any. How many weeks pregnant she is. Her TPAL is noted: T = number of pregnancies carried to term; P = premature deliveries; A = number of abortions, spontaneous or otherwise; L = the number of her living children. Here, too, are scrawled other important details. Are her membranes intact? If not, when did they rupture? How far apart are her contractions? What medication has she been given, and when? Is she a drug abuser? Is she HIV positive? What special conditions should be known? Diabetes? Preeclampsia? A previous cesarean section? What stage of labor is she in? What about the fetal heart tones? Changes in her cervix are noted as she progresses. All of this information, Sanskrit to the uninitiated, is scribbled in colored marking pens on a white board measuring approximately three feet high by five feet wide.

Crystal Mooney, twenty-nine, surrounded by friends in Room 16, is a long, thin woman with waist-length black hair and a narrow, canny face. Her chart notes her admission to a history of drug use. Let's say a very recent history. Chances are very, very good that her baby will be joining Timothy Edwards in the INCU across the hall, withdrawing for at least a couple of weeks, and catching up from being born too early, thanks to the drugs. Doesn't look like she'll be delivering for a couple of hours, at least.

Room 8 has Mary McGrath, blond and legally blind and twenty years old. It's her first baby, and two women friends—one completely blind—are with her. Her labor is in the early stages.

LaTonya Jordan, in Special Delivery, is thirteen, moving toward delivery, which looks like it won't happen for a while.

Her mother, a nurse points out, is dancing around the room, obviously stoned.

Marybeth O'Grady in Room 2 is twenty-six, and having her third child, the group is told. She is a part-time legal secretary, and her husband is in the room with her. No drugs during pregnancy. Her labor is progressing nicely.

Rounds completed, the knot of doctors, nurses and students disperses.

A resident checks in on a patient, a nurse goes into another room to read the heart tracings on another. Dr. Bissonnette walks through the double doors, returning to his office. The coast clear, everything momentarily under control, everyone else saunters into the coffee/supply room, drawn by the seductive smell of still-warm chocolate-chip cookies just brought in by a pretty medical student.

A half dozen or so green scrubs-suited people sit or stand around the chipped table, comparing notes, getting hits of camaraderie and mutual support along with the chocolate and sugar. The consensus is that OB/GYN is the perfect job for adrenaline junkies. And that the only way to stay wired enough for whatever fresh hell is racing—or awkwardly galumphing—toward them down the corridor is sugar, chocolate, and constant infusions of the strong coffee perpetually brewing on the Mr. Coffee to the right of the sink.

Working on 4NE's three-to-eleven P.M. shift is a job, and like some endless, baroquely plotted movie, there's no predicting the evening's unfolding story. At least with the women waiting downstairs in the Mother-Baby Unit, there are clues of what lies ahead. There's a severely obese woman down there who is likely to need a c-section when her baby is ready to emerge. A bored middle-class woman lies in her private room in the MBU, hoping that enforced bed rest will ensure the successful outcome of her in vitro fertilization pregnancy. A young blonde, still in her teens, has seriously high blood pressure. A young black girl, thirteen years old, is only six and a half months along, with no prenatal care. Her labor is tuning up, and she will soon need to come upstairs.

But who knows what will come through the swinging doors at the end of the hall on 4NE? A woman who has been beaten, and is miscarrying, perhaps? A private patient of one of the staff doctors?

Atop Marquam Hill with its dazzling view of the beautiful city built on both sides of the Willamette River, 4NE takes them all in. No woman is turned away because she can't pay for the delivery of her child. No woman is treated better than any other. Especially at first, each patient is addressed as "Miss" or "Mrs." Once a labor is going full strength, with its grunts and groans and screams leaking steadily from the labor room into the hallway, formality evaporates. It's "Push-push-push-*push*, Rita!" And "Give us another good *push*, LaWaunda!" And "You're doing a *wonderful* job, Kristi!"

A baby is born, sometimes the source of great celebration, sometimes causing only simple relief. Though the doctors and nurses may talk about it later, alone in the coffee/supply room beyond the nurses' station, their first concern is the child's well-being in the first hours of life outside the womb. The newcomer is carefully surveyed and rated, minutely if swiftly examined. Maybe there is a need for resuscitation, or for intravenous feeding. If the baby is premature, a stay in the Intermediate Neonatal Care Unit may be necessary until tiny lungs are sufficiently developed. The newborn's urine may be screened for drugs, a plan made for withdrawal from (sadly, frequently) crack cocaine.

Though at quick glance the nurses and the medical residents may appear glib, even uncaring, they are not. Between 200 and 250 babies are born each month on the fourth floor of North Hospital, and it isn't possible to get to know each delivering mother. To lose it, to break up over each sad thing that happens to a woman or her child, would render a doctor or nurse useless. Every case is special, each story unique. "The abruption in 10," "the HIV-positive in 8," "the twins in OR2" all have their special stories, their reasons for being the way they are, where they are.

Beyond the medical idiosyncrasies of each pregnancy and delivery, all the women come to 4NE for the same purpose: to have a baby. That seeming curtness, that impersonality, is in fact necessary for the doctor or nurse's survival. It is not a good idea, not a good idea at all, for a chronically exhausted resident to begin crying about the occasional baby who dies, or the newborn whose young life will surely soon be filled with indifferent care, or worse.

Doctors, nurses, and their patients: ships that pass in the night. For several hours, sometimes for days, they share one of life's most intensely intimate experiences, but when it's over, it's over. The patient goes home, usually with her baby. A month later she may, perhaps, recall some short lady in pale green pants and top holding her hand while a really great-looking bearded dude, drabbed out in the same unisex green getup, cut her *down there* and got her baby out.

The resident may, the next year, remember that terrific smile flashed by a blonde when handed her tiny premature son. (Was she the one with preeclampsia or the one whose boyfriend kept pacing so annoyingly?)

Indifferent doctors? Uncaring nurses? No. The signs of caring are all there. The steady, direct gaze into the patient's eyes as the resident tells her a cesarean section is needed to save the baby's life. The nurse holding the patient's hand—or foot—as she screams her way through another contraction. The simple, unspoken fact that the blood sport of obstetrics and gynecology has been chosen over more genteel specialties.

For the resident or nurse, making it through an evening shift can be exhilarating or heartbreaking or frustrating or educational or even, on occasion, boring. Borne bumpily aloft on strong coffee and weak jokes, each shift finally ends. The nurses (and even, eventually, the residents) return to their own lives, to echoing empty apartments or clamorous houses filled with long-suffering spouses and children.

It's a job.

According to The Board, Room 2's Marybeth O'Grady is twenty-six, and in the throes of producing her third child. What it doesn't say is that she is a blonde with a natural reddish shade that makes other women in the beauty salon grow briefly contemplative, then softly hiss, "Give me *that* color!"

Though not large, pacing out to some ten by twelve feet, Room 2 is one of the pleasantest of the labor and delivery rooms on 4NE. There's flowered wallpaper, a nice wooden chest of drawers. The big window has salmon-colored metal miniblinds. On the opposite wall is a large framed print of a Native American mother holding her little child.

At this particular moment in her life, Marybeth O'Grady is leaning back on her pillow in Room 2, those pale golden waves spread across the starched white case. Her husband, Dennis, a short, stocky red-haired man smelling faintly of fried food, holds her hand. After a nurse has completed her busy-work, Marybeth and Dennis O'Grady begin laughing. Neither is sure why they are laughing. Mostly, they are laughing in relief, happy that their old yellow Volvo station wagon made it up The Hill in time.

"That was close, my sweet, my pet, my chickadee," says the husband. "Perhaps next time we could plan on . . . oh, say, at least a two-hour labor?"

"Ah, you forget," replies the wife, frowning. "I'm getting my tubes tied right away—remember?"

"Oh, yes," says Dennis O'Grady, his freckled face growing swiftly serious.

"You still want to do it, don't you?" asks Marybeth. "We don't have to, you know. There's still time to change our mind."

"We've gone round and round on this, Marybeth. And we've talked and talked with Father Francis about it."

A Catholic couple, the O'Gradys have never had a child they've planned for. In fact, Patrick's impending arrival was what made her drop out of the University of Portland seven and a half years ago. Mary Elizabeth Wojcek had always dreamed of becoming a lawyer, and even after she met and fell in love with Dennis her first year at UP, she thought she could go to law school after she got her degree there. After a hasty wedding, they thought, Marybeth could just take a year or two off to care for Patrick, then (so the plan went), Dennis's mother would look after him while she went back to school. But then Dennis's mother got all forgetful, and it turned out she had Alzheimer's. Then Marybeth was pregnant with Molly.

A couple of years ago, Dennis—like hundreds of others—got laid off from Tektronix, where he was middle manage-ment. He's done some engineering consulting jobs since then, but they're erratic, and they've gotten fewer and fewer. And there have even been some nibbles from high-tech firms in

California's Silicon Valley. But Dennis's father died a couple of years ago, and they had to put Mother O'Grady in a nursing home. Now Marybeth's mother lives with them to help out with Patrick and Molly while Marybeth works half time as a legal secretary.

For the last year or so, Dennis has been working as shift manager at a drive-through burger joint out on Southeast Eighty-second. It's only thirty hours a week, with no bennies—certainly no medical insurance. And the pay is crummy, less than Marybeth's making with her part-time secretarial stuff. So far, with the $1,500 or so monthly take-home pay between them, the O'Gradys have been able to make ends meet, keeping up with the mortgage payments, feeding and clothing themselves and their children—and Marybeth's mother. But there's never anything left. Certainly nowhere near enough for private health insurance, which for their family of almost five would cost nearly $600 a month.

That's why Marybeth has been coming up The Hill, to the university's OB/GYN clinic for her prenatal checkups, why she is here tonight giving birth to her third child. And that is why, tomorrow, she will be having her tubes tied.

When Marybeth O'Grady arrived on L&D tonight, like all the other laboring women she was hooked up to a fetal heart-rate monitor. Two stretchable elastic belts were placed behind her back and around her swollen abdomen. One strap is connected to an ultrasound transducer. The other strap is connected to a pressure spring gauge, a device monitoring the presence, and sometimes the strength, of each uterine contraction. There are two reasons for putting Marybeth on the monitor. One is to learn whether she is truly in labor, by discerning the presence of regular defined uterine contractions, which should be occurring at the rate of three in a ten-minute period, with a slow onset, moving to a peak, then decelerating. The other reason she is on the FHR monitor is to get some idea of the well-being of the child within.

The fetal heart-rate monitor is an ultrasound machine, much like a radar or sonar, that emits sound waves, then detects reflections of those waves. In the process, it detects and spews out a long thin paper record, called a "strip," showing two thin graphlike lines. One line is the instantaneous fetal heart rate, a second-by-second recording; the other is a visible record of the mother's contractions. A healthy fetus will exhibit what's called a variability in the FHR—in normal terms ranging between 120 and 160 beats per minute—as well as good "beat-to-beat" variability. At any moment of checking the strip, it will vary, bouncing around, say, from 120 or 130 BPM to 140 BPM. And when the in utero baby is in generally good condition and active, turning and moving its arms and legs around, these movements are associated with accelerations in the fetal heart-rate tracing. These kinds of accelerations are good news: indications of the child's well-being, its freedom from disease, congenital malformation or oxygen starvation, and of a mature central nervous system. On the fetal heart-rate monitor machine, the baby's heartbeat sounds like a couple of coconut shells being whacked together: *pock! pock! pock!* The long paper strip swishes out of the machine, showing some unexplained decelerations, and this raises the question of whether the baby is in distress.

Dr. Gary Hoffman has just checked Marybeth's cervix a few minutes ago, and Third-Year Resident Julie Bouchard is having Medical Student Maggie Davis check out Marybeth's "lip"—the part of her cervix that hasn't yet given way. Student Nurse Heather Emmerich watches as Julie attaches an internal scalp electrode to the baby's head, deep inside Marybeth.

Med Student Maggie is three months pregnant. She watches all this, chewing gum in time to the music coming from the TV set. A *M*A*S*H* rerun shows Hawkeye examining a variety of feet. Then Julie Bouchard puts a long thin white plastic tube into Marybeth's vagina, working the end up against the baby's head inside. The device will literally record the child's electrocardiograph pattern. Holding very still, as she's been told, Marybeth asks if the procedure hurts the baby. Julie assures her that it doesn't.

As the minutes tick slowly by, Marybeth O'Grady's contractions continue, and as the baby's arrival draws nearer, she laughs nervously.

Dr. Gary Hoffman is fetched, and comes into Room 2. Maggie Davis, the pregnant medical student, injects Novocain into the perineum, then waits a minute or two. Then, she cuts an episiotomy with special scissors made for the purpose—

31

one blade with a blunted, curved end that can go inside the vagina, the other blade sharp. She makes a bloody slice through the area between the vagina and anus, enlarging the opening to facilitate the baby's emergence. So close, so close, and yet the baby doesn't come out. The decision is made to use the vacuum extractor to guide the infant out.

Basically the instrument, called a Mityvac, is a bell-shaped plastic cup measuring some four inches across the bell bottom. Seldom is the device used until the baby is well down into the mother's pelvis. And usually, as in Marybeth O'Grady's case, it is used to assist "outlet" delivery. Technically, the Mityvac is easier to use than forceps. Certainly, it is safer, though not without its own problems.

Forceps are used less and less nowadays, in part because cesarean sections are so much safer than in the past. (Incredible as it seems today, during the 1950s, many in the American obstetrical community regarded a forceps delivery as safer for the infant than normal labor.) Given the new understanding that forceps have been responsible for a high incidence of trauma and death for both mother and child, their use is being taught less in the country's medical schools. Yet, while the practice of "high forceps"—when they are used well up in the birth canal—is not often practiced, a forceps-assisted delivery is not uncommon. The Mityvac, the vacuum extractor, is not without its own dangers: Occasionally, for example, the baby's tender scalp is lacerated during the procedure, small hunks of skin ripped off.

It is a simple procedure, and for Marybeth O'Grady and her baby, it works quickly and well. Dr. Hoffman inserts the plastic bell into Marybeth's vagina, placing it against the child's head. Suction is applied, and the baby is—oh, so gently— pulled out of his mother.

A big, squalling, robust-looking boy weighing 9 pounds, 7.2 ounces. Immediately, he is named Joshua Matthew O'Grady. Joshua because that's the name of Marybeth's long-dead, much-loved grandfather. Matthew because she's always liked the name.

The resident and the medical student look the child over carefully, check his heart rate, evaluate his coloring, his muscle tone, his response to stimulation.

"Okay, Maggie," Dr. Gary Hoffman asks Maggie Davis. "What would you say his Apgar is?"

"Oh...I'd give him a seven...eight," says the pregnant med student, still chomping on her gum.

"Bingo," says Dr. Gary Hoffman. He turns to the new mother.

"Good work, Marybeth! This is a great-looking little kid you've got here!"

The system most frequently used to evaluate a newborn's transition to the outside world is the Apgar score. Named for its developer, Dr. Virginia Apgar, it is also an acronym: A for the infant's appearance, or color; P for pulse, or heart rate; G for grimace, or response to stimulation of aspiration; another A for activity, or muscle tone; and R for respirations.

With the Apgar, as in another kind of Olympics, a perfect score is a 10. For the Apgar's A, if the newborn's color is pale or blue, the score is 0; if only the extremities are blue or pale, the score is 1; and if the baby is totally pink, then 2 is the score. For the P, if the heart rate is not present at all, the score is 0; less than 100 beats per minute, it's a 1; greater than 100 beats per minute earns a 2. For the Apgar's G, the doctors try to "suck" the infant, suctioning its throat and nose, in the process checking the gag reflex. If the baby makes no grimace, the score is 0; if there is a grimace but no healthy protest, the score is 1; if the response is a vigorous crying, the maximum score of 2 is awarded. For the Apgar's second A, representing activity or muscle tone, a flaccid newborn is scored 0, some muscle tone in the limbs receiving a 1, and good flexion, active moving about with good muscle tone, is rated 2. Finally, the R: The baby's respirations are rated 0 if absent; 1 if slow, irregular, or shallow; and receive a 2 if good, regular, and deep, with crying when the baby meets the earth's cool air—and with cruelly poking, prodding strangers after months of warmth in the mother's womb.

Although imperfect, the Apgar score is probably as good an indicator there is of fetal well-being immediately following birth. It may or may not be a reflection of the asphyxia—oxygen deprivation—that sometimes follows labor. Low Apgars can result from several causes. In the current legal climate, replete with eager lawyers doing the bidding of disappointed new parents who didn't get their guaranteed perfect baby, low Apgars are often believed to result from birth injury. From somebody doing something wrong. The fact is that many injuries suffered by newborns have taken place before birth, as a result of neurological "insults," in medical parlance—often drugs the mother shared with her unborn child. And a low Apgar score may be the result of severe congenital abnormalities, the 2 percent to 4 percent of unexplained birth defects that simply happen in a world that is (and always has been) less than perfect.

Down the hall, the clock above the nurses' station says that it's 1903, 7:03 P.M. Unheard in the white noise that's part of 4NE's work life, a gracefully bulbous-looking contraption, a Harley-Davidson motorcycle, reminiscent of police bikes from fifties movies, roars up to the parking lot behind North Hospital. It stops, and deafeningly loud mufflers are silenced. A biker and his woman dismount, both with some awkwardness, given the size of their bellies. The woman, whose name is Harriet Grackle, is very pregnant. Herman Grackle, who everyone calls "Animal," has a huge beer gut. On his old leather vest, among many patches, is a frayed one reading: LOUD PIPES SAVE LIVES.

"This time," says the woman. "This is it. This time I *know* I'm in labor, Animal."

"Harriet," says her husband. "Baby. It's okay. You ain't in labor, we just come back as many times as it takes." He leans over in the soft April gloaming to give her a smooch on the cheek. Hand in hand, the couple lumbers to the door leading to the elevator to the Labor and Delivery Department. It is the third time they have ridden their ancient Panhead from North Portland in the last ten days.

Upstairs, First-Year Resident Tracey Delaplain has just sent Louise Bradshaw back home. Louise is very thin, except for her in utero twins. From behind, as she walks slowly down the hall toward the swinging doors, Louise doesn't look pregnant at all. But from the front, it's a different story. Louise complains of feeling tired all the time. Of wanting to do nothing but sleep. Something Tracey can understand, being six months along herself.

Filipinas Mugas Cox, thirty-nine, rounds the corner to see if Marybeth O'Grady has vacated Labor Room 2, to check if it's ready to be prepared for the next occupant. "Fili," as everyone calls her, is popular with the nurses and doctors she works with, appreciated as she cleans the beds, restocks the rooms, mops the floors, and performs the dozen other jobs assigned to her as a hospital aide. It's hard work, harder than anything Fili has done before in her life. And these days, with the threat of AIDS, working directly with the blood of others is dangerous work as well.

Right away, when the tiny, thin Filipino woman comes on her three-to-eleven-P.M. shift, she dons the blue or green scrubs, the uniform that makes her, at first glance, indistinguishable from the other workers on 4NE. When she scrubs out and prepares one of the two operating rooms at the end of the hall, she puts on a disposable mask and hair covering, helping to keep the ORs as sterile as possible. Right away, at the beginning of her shift, Fili usually checks the warmer, where they keep the baby blankets and the thermal blankets and the various solutions and the distilled water. She restocks what's needed from the supply cart kept in the room between the hall and the staff bathroom. Fili checks the fetal monitor belts, making sure they're available.

After a woman delivers and is transported downstairs to the Mother-Baby Unit, Fili enters the empty labor room, with its warm, fresh-baked smells of fecundity, and readies it for the next go-round. She strips the bed of sheets, pillow, and blankets. Then, with a gallon of water disinfectant solution, her small hands protected by latex gloves, Fili scrubs down the vinyl-upholstered mattress, then mops the floor of its bodily fluids: blood, perhaps, and amniotic fluid, and, sometimes, excrement. She replenishes the labor room's supplies, bringing in surgical gloves, linens, the Betadine antiseptic solution, and remakes the bed.

It is also part of Fili Cox's job to weigh the placenta after a birth, and to clean and sterilize the instruments used during the delivery—chores that differentiate her job from that of the housekeepers. On weekends, there is no housekeeper, and the nurses sometimes must lend a hand with the floor mopping and trash removal. They don't complain. It's all part of everyone's job, they tell Fili.

This hard, hard work, this physically exhausting labor, is not at all what Filipinas Mugas Cox thought she would be doing at this point of her life.

Her early life, back in the Philippines, was luxurious. There were always maids to do the housework, and, as one of seven children of a coconut plantation owner—in pre-Marcos days the mayor of San Policarpo, a town in the eastern part of Samar—Fili was adored and indulged. After completing high school, Fili went to work in a big department store in Manila, selling Max Factor cosmetics, remaining unmarried, enjoying this work for fourteen years until her father urged her to return to school. Unwilling to undertake a full university education, Fili chose a two-year midwifery course.

Part of Fili's midwifery training was to assist in twenty deliveries, to deliver a score of babies on her own, and then to deliver ten infants in a home setting, away from a hospital. Unlike in the United States, in Philippine hospitals midwives are not permitted to examine patients internally, nor to suture—sew up—tears in the perineum that may occur during a delivery. Instead, in case of a bad laceration, patients are taken to hospitals for the perineal repairs, then sent back home.

By the time she took the midwives' board exams, Fili had decided to go to America, to see what living there might be like. Visiting relatives in Southern Oregon, she met and married an American railroad worker. She was thirty-one. Four days after their wedding, Fili's new husband was laid off from his job. Soon the couple moved to Oklahoma, where they lived for six years and where he worked in the booming oil industry. Fili found a job she loved, in a hospital looking after the newborns. Childless herself, she found joy in making bonnets and booties for her small charges.

When Fili and Jackie Cox moved to Portland in 1986, she applied for a job on Pill Hill. While waiting to be called, she worked at a nursing home. Finding the heavy lifting too much for her, Fili became certified as a "medication aide." When

OHSU finally offered her a job as an aide in the Labor and Delivery Department, she knew it would be hard, physical work. But she knew, too, that working at OHSU would be less depressing than at the nursing home, where the most she earned was $4.00 an hour. OHSU was offering her $4.65 to start.

Fili's husband is a truck driver now, with his own truck. He's gone so much, though, sometimes for many nights at a time, so they share a house with some of Fili's cousins from the Philippines. One of her cousins was a pediatrician back home, but she hasn't passed the boards here, and so she works at the hospital as an EKG technician.

Sometimes the work gets kind of tiresome. But the doctors here at the hospital are nice. They introduce themselves, and they don't say, "I'm Dr. So-and-So." They just say their first name. It's really busy and hard sometimes, and sometimes you wish you don't work here. But that happens with any kind of job.

Maybe she'll go back to school, Fili thinks, maybe take nursing. The one thing Fili likes best about her job is helping these mothers. Once in a while, she kind of wishes she were the one delivering the babies. But she knows she's helping these mothers to deliver safely.

Knowing that, it helps her in her daily chores. Especially if it's real busy, Fili gets worried. Like if there are three ladies waiting, and she can see someone is very uncomfortable and she thinks, *Oh! This one is delivering in the hallway!* She always tries to clean the room as fast as she can and make sure no one will deliver in the hallway! It's hard work cleaning the rooms, and dangerous coming into contact with blood. But even though Fili doesn't get to see the babies being born, she knows she's a part of the miracle.

CHAPTER TWO

The City of Roses

OVER THE DECADES, MANY new Portlanders have arrived in the city without job prospects, knowing nobody. Pulled toward this state, drawn to this city, they may come for one reason, then remain for other, quite different ones.

Despite the difficulties of her job, despite wishing (once in a while) she was the one delivering the babies on 4NE, Fili Cox loves living here. Following his job-seeking American tour in the mid-1970s, Dr. E. Paul Kirk had no trouble choosing Portland as the place to finish rearing his family. One reason that Dr. Kirk's chief of obstetrics lives in Portland, and works at OHSU, is because of his dismay at California's Proposition 13's decimation of that state's school system. A certain handsome resident is here, and will stay here, because his firstborn, a SIDS casualty, is buried here. A red-haired chief resident went to medical school with the head of the OB/GYN residency program, and so looked at doing her residency here. Then she and her husband found a wonderful old house on a generous hunk of farmland, smack in the middle of nearby Sauvie Island.

Portland, Oregon, is a city long celebrated for its charms,

over the years frequently cited by national magazines for its "livability." Its reputation, in fact, reached such heights back in the 1960s and 1970s that a conscious campaign was mounted, a movement reaching deeply into official governmental levels. Jealously protecting the state's chaste, unsullied condition, Oregonians nonetheless welcomed the tourist dollar. Out-of-staters were encouraged to visit (and, of course, to spend lots of money), and then to return from whence they came. DON'T CALIFORNICATE OREGON went one popular slogan, stuck onto thousands of automobile bumpers, sticking it as well to the state's neighbors to the south.

The city of Portland, its official population just under 400,000, serves a metropolitan area of more than a million people, most of whom shrug amiably when asked about the seeming-constant rain, which lasts from October through April, with frequent damp reminders during the other months. The city sits some eighty miles from the Pacific Ocean beaches, which form the state's westernmost border, stretching from the bottom corner of Washington State to California's top corner. No one owns the beach. Or, more precisely, everyone owns the beach, thanks to a visionary governor named Oswald West, who pushed through legislation back in 1913, making the ocean beaches public property. And Portland is equidistant from the slopes of Mount Hood, with skiing potential that draws vacationers from other parts of the country.

Portlanders—typically, those transplanted from New York City, say, or Houston, or Los Angeles—boast that their chosen city has a small-town feel, with relatively unpolluted air, but with big-city amenities. Portland has its own opera company and symphony orchestra, a punk-music venue or two, and a startlingly vivid live theater scene. A well-developed library system is run by Multnomah County, its splendid colonnaded central library open seven days a week. Road company Broadway shows make the city a regular stop between the larger cities of Seattle and San Francisco, as do comedy acts like Jay Leno and George Carlin. Other popular nationally and internationally known performers—ranging from Luciano Pavarotti to Johnny Mathis, all the way down to The Butthole Surfers (or up, depending on your musical tastes)—can count on a healthy Portland turnout.

The temperature seldom dips below freezing, and because of the rain, lawns remain green year-round. Rhododendrons grow as high as trees, and rosebushes abound, blooming from May well into the autumn months. "You can't kill a rosebush here," insist the region's proud-but-modest gardeners, waving aside compliments on their extravagant blooms.

The city, in fact, glories in its reputation as the Rose City, and annually indulges in an orgy of civic self-celebration called the Rose Festival, reigned over by a Rose Queen selected from a comely bevy of teenaged girls who strut their nubile stuff before a population swelled by thousands of visitors, including naval fleets from several countries.

While the cost of living per se is not dramatically lower than that of comparable American cities, less than $100,000 will still buy a splendid prewar house in a good neighborhood. ("A *mansion*! A *mansion*!" freshly defected San Franciscans have been heard gushing into long-distance telephone lines, describing their newly acquired homes. "With a *fireplace*! And *oak floors*! And *leaded glass windows*!")

Yet, the economic recession that afflicted much of America in the early 1980s hit the state of Oregon with powerful force. With its economy largely lumber based, and that industry especially hard hit, the state's unemployment rate has skyrocketed. Suddenly, miraculously, Oregon lost much of its official and unofficial coolness toward outsiders. (Some, of course, insisted that they had always regarded the attitude as downright snobbishness.) Tourism began to be vigorously promoted, sans the sniffy implication that a welcome *can* be overstayed. Industry was aggressively sought by governors and mayors, who proffered tax incentives, fat worms on hooks dangled before the noses of Japanese and German companies which just might build factories that "meant jobs," as the phrase went. (Even, grumped some, to those once-shunned industries of the "polluting" sort.)

With an economy only partially recovered, coupled with a population rise, Oregon (and especially Portland) has by now acquired most of the predictable problems of a late-twentieth-century American metropolis.

As befits a sizable American city in these times, Portland has a thriving crime rate. It is a veritable paradise for the

41

career criminal, asserts one not-terribly-conservative county judge, who knows that the sentences he imposes will never be fully served in a state with woefully inadequate jail space. Some, city-proud Portlanders of long standing, try to convince themselves that the statistics lugubriously reported on the evening news and in the morning newspaper simply reflect a citizenry that *reports* crime more often. An egg thrown at a neighbor's garage by a cranky prepubescent kid is, they say, stirred in with other "crime" statistics.

But as the days, months, and years wear on, even the blindest, even the most optimistic, must admit the obvious: Portland has a serious drug problem. Police raids on crack houses are reported with disheartening regularity on the nightly news. The Bloods and the Crips, juvenile gangs based in Los Angeles, have become part of the picture—even creating a ruckus, loaded guns and all, one Saturday night at the Rose Festival Fun Center. A small but active contingent of Nazi skinhead gangs has made its presence known—with, among other acts, unprovoked beatings of nonwhites, and, once, a particularly vicious baseball-bat beating murder of an Ethiopian immigrant. The increased volume of rapes and muggings, of robberies and murders, places the City of Roses well within the country's champion cities for incidence of violent crimes per capita.

The area's economy has recovered, but in ways that bleakly underscore the widening chasm between the haves and the have-nots. Near the river, in Northwest Portland, close at hand to shelters for the city's homeless, old factory lofts are being cunningly "reinterpreted" into trendy "living spaces" for a growing class of the semiwealthy: studio apartments renting for $900-plus monthly. Northwest Twenty-third Avenue, once a cheery melange of thrift shops and arty boutiques, has dumped the former for the latter and become a favorite boulevard for hordes of strolling Yuppies and their nattily togged young.

Yet, for many, little has changed. Many who once had jobs still have none. Mortgages once kept up have defaulted. Thousands of people are now homeless, many of them young families who can no longer afford to pay rent. More people have joined the public-assistance rolls. Men and women who once earned very good salaries, plus benefits, at places like Tektronix and Georgia Pacific and Weyerhaeuser, flip burgers and take orders at Burger King and McDonald's. (And find that they're scheduled for less than full-time hours, to spare their thrifty employers the expense of providing benefits.)

Not qualifying for Medicaid, nor receiving medical benefits through their work, and unable, with their minimum-wage jobs, to afford their own health insurance, these people have become the New Indigent. And while they buy lottery tickets every week, hoping that their bad luck will break, they pray that nothing goes wrong, not with themselves, with their spouses, or with their kids. And they deliver their babies at OHSU.

2125: 9:25 P.M.

In the Exam Room, Harriet Grackle is ready to scream. Once again, she is not in labor. Once again, she is being told to go home. Being this pregnant is the pits. She has a four-year-old son. Not Animal's kid, but a souvenir of her wilder days before they met. By the time Tommy was born, they'd already gotten married, and everyone assumes he's the father. The way Animal Grackle looks at it, Tommy's his son. End of discussion. Period. Animal, he's like that.

You wouldn't know it to look at her now, but Harriet had a brief career as a topless dancer, a stripper if you want to be real honest about it. For four or five years there—not as Harriet Louise Grondahl, of course, but as "Trisha Darling"—she worked at Magic a Go-Go, down on Northwest Fourth in Old Town. Night after night. She wasn't exactly a hooker, but if she went off with a customer and they did it and he happened to give her fifty or one hundred bucks afterward, she didn't exactly hand the money back. That is how she ended up with Tommy. Harriet can't remember how many abortions she's had. Somehow, when she found out she was pregnant nearly five years ago with Tommy, she decided she'd had enough, already. God only knows who the father was. And what difference does it make now, anyway?

And then one Thursday night this grubby bunch of bikers

43

stomps into Magic a Go-Go, when Harriet's filling in for Mary Ann Kilgore (a.k.a. "Bambi"), just gyrating away a mile a minute in her Trisha Darling getup, red-sequined bikini, twirling tassels and all. The whole time the bikers are in there, this Animal guy is looking at her like WHAT ARE YOU DOING HERE? Anyway, he takes a real shine to her, and she goes home with him, and everything is different. Everything.

Next thing she knows, Animal is taking her away from all this, like they used to say in the movies. He doesn't mind about her being pregnant with some other guy's baby, and he doesn't care that she's a stripper and that she used to get paid for doing other stuff, sometimes. He thinks she's just beautiful and wonderful and he wants to marry her and take care of her and Tommy and to have another kid or two.

The erstwhile Trisha Darling just wishes to hell she could have this baby tonight. She puts her underpants back on and her capri pants and her red flower-printed sleeveless maternity top. Animal zips up the back for her. Then Harriet and Herman "Animal" Grackle leave the Exam Room. Hand in hand, they begin their slow journey back down the hall, to the elevator, down to the first floor. Back in the parking lot, they strap on their helmets, remount the Harley, and roar off, back to North Portland.

Down in the third floor's Mother-Baby Unit, a couple of rooms down from still-stoned red-haired Cammie Edwards, lies Lily Pratt, who has never even smoked a marijuana cigarette. Despite her nightie of lace-trimmed pink plissé, even under the covers she is enormous, a benign mountain of a woman. Lily is thirty-five, and her weight before becoming pregnant was 497 pounds. Now, lying on her back, her 155-pound husband perched birdlike in the chair beside her, Lily couldn't be happier—or more scared. For years she has been told that she would never bear a child. Then, without warning, something happened, some miracle transpired, and Lily was pregnant. Oh, happy day!

So happy is this woman, in fact, that every time she speaks of this astonishing thing, she begins to weep. Scott David is the name already assigned to her boy child, she says. Scotty, for short. For Scotty she will lose weight again, begin to look like a normal woman. Scotty will not have to be embarrassed by his mother.

For now, though, there's the delivery to get through.

Lily Pratt is having her baby on Pill Hill because, as a nearly five-hundred-pound *primigravida*—first-time mother-to-be—she's regarded as high-risk. Back home in the Pratts' hometown of Gold Beach, on the southern Oregon coast, no obstetrician worth his yearly malpractice-insurance premium would accept her as a patient. While not unheard-of, it is unusual for a woman of Lily's weight to be able to accomplish a "normal" vaginal delivery. Through the heavy layers of fat, it is well-nigh impossible to get a decent ultrasound picture of the fetus, and so its condition, despite other tests, on some levels must remain mysterious. Cutting through the mounds of abdominal fatty tissue for a cesarean section will not only be surgically very difficult, but could also be life-threatening. Fat is disinclined to heal easily, and the possibility of postoperative complications is very strong.

Because of her obesity, it hasn't been possible to adequately follow the well-being of Lily's child. Nor has there been the normal measure of maternal weight gain in pregnancy. Because of her gestational diabetes, and because of some indications through ultrasound testing, the belief is that the child already weighs ten or eleven pounds—a huge baby to emerge from any mother, even one of Lily's size. A fetus that large can be susceptible to birth trauma, which would prevent a normal vaginal delivery. Also it has not been possible to do an amniocentesis to check the baby's lung maturity.

The hope is that by inducing Lily's labor, a number of these problems can be sidestepped, and that delivery by cesarean section will be less likely. However, many times inductions go awry, with the mother having to be sectioned anyway because an adequate labor can't be accomplished. Lily also has what's called "evolving preeclampsia," high blood pressure; once such a diagnosis is made, it's necessary to proceed in the direction of delivery.

In itself, obesity is a horrendous risk factor. For a number of reasons, it is especially so for cesarean sections. Even in women whose obesity is much less severe than Lily's, there

45

is the *pannus* to deal with. The pannus is the abdominal extension of the belly, an overgrowth that flops down toward the crotch—in other words, a man's twenty-years' worth of beer belly on a woman. And if you think the fetus is in distress, it may take a long, long time to get through all that, and to bring the baby out.

In a cesarean section, where do you go with this? As the doctor, do you go above the huge overlapping pannus, cutting through a large amount of it, in order to get to the uterus and the child? Or, using clips, do you literally pull the pannus back up, away from the region of the crotch and the lower uterine segment, so that you can make an incision? Usually, the incision has to be made in the reflection of the skin—a bad, bad area for yeast growth and other normal skin flora. Often, this area is already reddened, eroded from chronic irritation from hanging over the skin below. It's not at all a good place to place an incision. But if you go in over the pannus, then you risk having to cut through a massive layer of fat that is poorly vascularized and that is not going to heal well, creating a dreadful risk for postoperative complications.

There are also serious problems in how to close the wound. Should multiple drains be left in? Should the wound be left open for two or three days so that the fluid from the fat can be drained? There's almost a guarantee that, once sectioned, Lily Pratt would have a terrible wound infection in the subcutaneous fat. Inside, from the area of the fascia, probably five to seven inches would have to be laid open and bared. She would probably be incapable of caring for it herself. It would, in fact, probably take four or five months for this wound to heal completely, even if a serious infection did not set in it.

From the standpoint of the anesthesiologist, someone this seriously obese presents great difficulties as well. An epidural would be the safest kind of anesthesia, yet it's nearly impossible to find the landmarks, to locate specifically where the needle should go in. It's difficult to find a spinal needle long enough to insert correctly in the region you want it. A general anesthetic, putting the patient out completely for a c-section, can be problematical as well, since there would be difficulty ventilating her. She is at increased risk for aspiration, and for cardiac problems during the procedure itself.

While she is hardly aware of the details of her risky delivery to come, Lily Pratt knows some of this, and she has been very grateful for the excellent care she knows she has been receiving from Chief Resident Nicholas Abrudescu during her regular clinic visits. But Dr. Abrudescu is on vacation and her care has fallen to the other residents.

Lily talks on and on, and her husband, David, smiles with transcendent sweetness at the wife he calls "Ma." David is a millworker. He was laid off a couple of months ago, Lily tells her roommate, a tiny Asian woman who watches the television, looking over at Lily every minute or so, nodding and smiling and not comprehending a word of what is being said. Lately, while he looks for a real job, David has been working part time at a Safeway store, bagging groceries. Lily speaks for them both, as is evidently their custom.

When Lily Pratt—Lillian Patricia Parsons then—was in the second grade, she already weighed 125 pounds. The women in Lily's family have always been big. So far, Lily's the biggest one in her family, but they're all big. She's the youngest of eight kids, and everyone still treats her like the baby. Probably always will.

It's a horrible life, just awful, being this fat. But like they say, there's someone for everyone. When Lily met David Pratt nine years ago, she was plenty big. In fact, on their wedding day eight years ago, she weighed 430 pounds.

After Lily and David had been married for three years, she got down to 165 pounds—and she kept it off for three years, too. And then it all came back. It was just like she'd learned to ski from a book, and suddenly found herself on an icy mountain slope. You have to have real skills to deal with everything. It was just too much for her to handle, with everything she was doing.

For a while, Lily worked as an accountant. That was when she was thinner. She worked for a big hotel, as their accounts-receivable person. They trained her and everything, and she liked it. Then the weight was coming back, and she quit. She couldn't fit in chairs very well, and this thing was always in her head: What if the chairs in this room or that one all had arms, and she couldn't fit in them?

Lily was going to nursing school at a community college full time, getting straight A's, too. She just started eating. It was just like she was still big and fat inside, even though she was skinny on the outside. And the weight came right back on, more than 250 pounds. In a way, it just seemed like Lily was doing it on purpose after a while. The more she eats, when she's this big, then she doesn't have to go out of the house and face anything. It sounds weird, but maybe, Lily thinks, she's just kind of trying to shut herself out from life. If she's big and fat, she doesn't have to go out. Not that she doesn't shop some, not for clothes so much, but for other stuff, household items and the like. But it's not fun. People look. It's almost like racial prejudice, the way people act toward fat people.

Lily's a nice person, she knows that. And David loves her. He never mentions her weight. When Lily talks about it, he always says, *"Oh, Ma!"* He just thinks she's crazy to take on the way she does about it. But Lily worries about it for her health, not just her appearance. This baby coming is really a godsend. It's really helped Lily start getting it all under control. She got gestational diabetes with the pregnancy, and Dr. Abrudescu put her on a strict diet, and she's lost thirty-five pounds since January.

After the baby comes, maybe she'll join Overeaters Anonymous. One of Lily's cousins, the one who's a nurse, has been going there and she recommends it. Lily's gone to Weight Watchers, but she worries that they'll have those little teeny scales that don't weigh people Lily's size. Her scales at home go up to 500. Lily's never been that fat. But close, real close.

Down the hall of the Mother-Baby Unit, a woman screams, her labor starting to tune up.

"Gee," says Lily Pratt to the woman in the bed across the room from her. "I hope I don't do *that!*"

As Lily Pratt talks of little Scott and her plans for him, across the hall primigravida Hilary Blanchard glares out the window of her room. She's been here for three weeks already, and is likely to be here for at least another two months. The reason, the only reason, Hilary's been sentenced to week after boring week in this dump of a hospital, languishing in Pill Hill's Mother-Baby Unit, is because her doctor, Philip Patton, heads up OHSU's in vitro fertilization program. And if it weren't for IVF, the high school art teacher and her dentist husband wouldn't even be holding on to this pregnancy. If she can just hang on for a couple more months, they'll get a baby out of the deal.

Life, Hilary knows by now, isn't fair. It was more than thirty years ago when her own mother was having trouble getting pregnant, going through one miscarriage after another. So, in accordance with the obstetrical custom of the day, her mother was put on a regimen with a "miracle" drug called diethylstilbesterol. We know now about DES, and about the resultant girl babies called "DES daughters."

It will probably take years to sort out exactly how DES affected the reproductive systems of the children whose mothers took the drug. Yet there seems little doubt that the effects are significant.

What Hilary Blanchard apparently got from her mother's use of DES (besides her existence on this earth) was an "incompetent cervix," one that cannot stay sufficiently closed to contain a baby for the full term of forty weeks. And there's something wrong with her fallopian tubes, too.

So, one morning last August, the technicians at OHSU's fertility clinic surgically fetched out a half-dozen eggs from one of Hilary Blanchard's ovaries. Placed in a Petri dish, the eggs were fertilized with sperm freshly donated by her husband. They were carefully watched over, and those that "took" were frozen for possible later implantation. Hilary had the ready-to-go pre-embryos, called "zygotes," implanted in her uterus, but the first try didn't take. Two months later, the procedure was repeated. Later, when she threatened to miscarry, Dr. Patton performed an operation called a *cerclage,* gathering up the outer edges of her cervix, like a ribbon threaded through the top of a pouch, to keep labor from beginning.

Yet even this surgery was insufficient to ensure a successful, full-term pregnancy for Hilary. Probably because of the DES her mother took, Hilary has an extremely small T-shaped uterus. Given her incompetent cervix, without the cerclage she would doubtless have prematurely dilated before term—miscarrying, losing her baby. Even with the cerclage, the purse string that Dr. Patton threaded through her cervix, the centimeter or so that the cervix had dilated has completely evaporated, and the cervix has become a paper-thin piece of tissue. Right now, all that separates Hilary's child from the outside of the womb is the stitch Dr. Patton made. It was decided that complete bed rest would be the safest route. In the hospital, at that, where Dr. Patton could keep an eye on her.

This was not good news to Hilary Blanchard. Not at all. She and her husband, Richie, live in Central Oregon, and it wasn't exactly convenient to move to Portland, 150-odd miles distant, for such a long, uncertain time. Oh well, Hilary and Richie would just have to make the best of a rotten situation. They would just pretend that Hilary wasn't in a hospital at all. Certainly not in this one, with its bare walls and dingy colors, and (let's not mince words here) the kinds of women who *have* to have their babies here. Given any choice, the couple agreed, Hilary would be cozily tucked into Good Sam or Emanuel, with a decent meal served after the ordeal of birth—and a decent wine—a carpet on the floor and at least a graphic or two on the walls.

When life hands you a lemon, you make lemonade, right? And if they are going to have to *pay* for Hilary to stay here, they're going to get their money's worth, by God. Hilary is going to get a massage, daily. And as for the food, well, she'll just have her meals catered several nights a week, brought in from this great little place in Northwest Portland called Briggs & Crampton. (The meals are all garnished with edible fresh flowers. Cute, huh?)

Richie brought in some of Hilary's silk screens from their bedroom and put them up on a room divider. They brought her framed print of "The Unicorn in Captivity" tapestry. Always—always, this is important!—there will be fresh flowers in the room. And Perrier water. Hilary's hairdresser will come in every week to razor-cut her short, chic golden blond "do." And when she rings for a nurse, one had damned well better

50

show up. Right now. Dr. Patton—Philip to the Blanchards—comes by daily, continually assuring Hilary that it's fine to despise him for putting her through all this. I mean, we are talking *bored* here. Capital B, B-O-R-E-D-O-M.

Observing all this, the MBU nurses have taken to referring to Dr. Philip Patton as "Philippe," and to his patient as "Our Little Princess." (What in God's name is the deal with that weird unicorn picture, anyway?) And while they aren't usually excited by her suggestion that they finish up what she can't eat from her Briggs & Crampton repast, one night, the pretty blond nurse and the heavy charge nurse, rather than flipping their usual coin, took turns spooning mouthfuls of Our Little Princess's left-over (but untouched) chocolate mousse garnished with the delicate petals of violets.

CHAPTER THREE

Day 2: Tuesday, April 12

("Nobody is guaranteed a perfect baby," says the residency program head.)

1455: 2:55 P.M.

DR. MARK NICHOLS, HEAD of Pill Hill's OB/GYN residency program, sits at his desk, poring (again) over the work schedules of his residents. There's really no way to work this out—not so that everyone is happy, anyway. One of the residents is taking time off, and another is about to. The first one has been spending time in the Midwest with her sick mother, who finally died. The other has learned that her mother—in Florida—has cancer, with scant weeks to live. There's just no way Dr. Nichols can cover their absences by adding to the burden of the already overworked residents: They have to sleep *sometime*. The solution is obvious, one that will be unpopular with his colleagues. The doctors on the departmental faculty will have to fill in, "taking call" more in order to compensate.

Just as surely as people get born, they die. You can predict the time for one, maybe. But not the other.

Predestiny. The way his mother tells it, when Mark Nichols was born back in the early fifties, his grandmother responded to the news of her daughter's firstborn with: "Mark David . . . M.D.! Oh, he's going to be a doctor, huh?"

Early on, it was drilled into him by his father, a county administrator, that people "should make a contribution to society"—a phrase he and his sister and two brothers heard a lot as they were growing up in Santa Rosa, an hour's drive from San Francisco. Their mother, a homemaker (whose skills were probably underutilized in those less enlightened days, he now believes) joined in encouraging her oldest child to go into some aspect of science that would serve others. In high school, he met with different doctors, went on hospital rounds to see what that life was all about. He did well in school, getting his undergraduate degree at the University of California at Davis, and medical school just kept seeming like a good idea. And so he attended medical school at UC Davis, finishing in 1979.

Personality probably has a lot to do with why doctors choose their specialties, Dr. Nichols thinks, and he probably has the right sort for obstetrics. As a second-year med student, he was told to get involved in some community-based health care program, and decided to attend Lamaze classes. In the class was a woman whose merchant marine husband was always away, and who was having their third child. Perhaps it was the thrill of combat, but the young medical student volunteered to be her labor coach. (Certainly he wasn't thinking of becoming an OB/GYN, uh-uh.)

Then he took a human sexuality class, then some other OB-related activities, again, never really meaning to become an OB/GYN, no sir. Like most third-year students going through all the rotations, he pictured himself as an internal medicine doctor, then as a general surgeon, then an orthopedist. Then he went through the OB rotation, and it was wonderful. He got a lot of positive feedback from people he worked with. He approached patients well, they told him. It was, he finally admitted, a good fit.

Dr. Nichols came to Oregon Health Sciences University to do his four-year residency in OB/GYN, planning to enter private practice when the residency was completed in 1983. Pill Hill's OB/GYN chairman at the time was Leon Speroff, with whom the resident became friendly, even delivering the chairman's wife's baby. Dr. Speroff encouraged Mark Nichols to consider remaining at OHSU as a member of the depart-ment's staff. Working with Dr. Speroff appealed to him, but the chairman was probably moving to Cleveland's Case West-ern Reserve. If the department, under a new chairman, were to change drastically, that appeal would be gone. But the Case Western job was offered to someone else, not to Dr. Speroff, and Dr. Mark Nichols agreed to sign on the dotted line. But in the end, Dr. Speroff did go to Case Western, taking with him a number of the OHSU staff.

With Pill Hill's OB/GYN faculty decimated, at a new all-time low, Dr. Nichols thought he should stick around just to help out. Eighteen months passed before Acting Chairman Dr. E. Paul Kirk was appointed to the permanent position. (It was a natural, of course. Dr. Kirk had for some years been program chairman, with a lot of other administrative functions within the department, including acting as chairman during the times when Dr. Speroff was out of town.) But during the whole search, Dr. Nichols was very nervous: What if they hired some Attila the Hun? But Paul is great, thinks Dr. Nichols. A wonderful man.

Dr. Mark Nichols's official title is Assistant Professor, the Associate Program Director for Residency Training. As an assistant professor, he teaches the residents and the medical students. A not-so-implied implication is that research is ac-complished at the same time.

As an obstetrician/gynecologist with private patients, Dr. Nichols basically charges the community's going rate—$1,800 for the total OB package, including all prenatal care, the de-livery, and a postpartum office visit. In private practice, Dr. Nichols would probably take home about 70 percent of that, the rest going to pay overhead. Another way private patients get dinged is with their hospital fees; the charge for a hospital bed at OHSU is higher than anywhere else in Portland. In order to stay profitable, so the reasoning goes (offsetting the expense of indigent patient care), the payers—the insurance companies, the sources of public assistance, and others—must be charged higher rates than elsewhere. Not that they all pay what's asked. Huge numbers of people here do nothing but do battle with insurance companies.

It's necessary for Dr. Nichols to keep a thriving private

practice going, both in order to help keep the department afloat and to keep his own salary comparable, if not competitive, with what he might make in full-time private practice. With all the hours he's working up here, he knows he could be making a lot more money out on his own. That's true of all the faculty. He's paid $90,000 a year, with some possible bonuses at year's end. From talking to friends from residency days, Dr. Nichols knows he could make twice that, easy.

Malpractice? People think Dr. Nichols doesn't have to bother about it. Maybe he doesn't have to worry about paying the premiums, but in fact he has lots more exposure to malpractice than his private-practice colleagues. For instance, next month—May—he'll be attending labor and delivery, splitting that duty with another staff doctor. The two of them will ultimately be responsible for every baby born on Pill Hill during the month of May—that's maybe 250. So statistically, Dr. Nichols will be responsible for 125 deliveries. Of those 125, he will be present at maybe 10 percent of them. He'll be there during perhaps 20 percent of the cesarean sections and the forceps deliveries. The other 80 percent are probably going to do fine.

But say in five years, one of the babies has developed a learning disability? If they go back into the records to find out who was medically legally responsible, than it's going to be yours truly. So he has much more exposure to malpractice than his buddies out there in private practice. At least he doesn't have to worry about the liability, since ORS 30.260–30.300, the state torts claims act, limits malpractice lawsuit claims to $200,000 "per event," and sets a limit of $500,000 for the total number of claims per event.

This notion of the guaranteed perfect baby is insidious. The fact is that 2 percent to 4 percent of all pregnancies are going to end in some kind of congenital malformation. That's just the baseline. What causes this percentage of risk is hard to understand. A lot of it is "environmental"—medical bullshit for not knowing the explanation. But that's the baseline incidence, okay? Why has it come to pass that someone has to be responsible for that?

It seems to Dr. Nichols that when he was growing up, if a child had a birth defect, it was just accepted. It was considered unfortunate, tragic, and there was an attempt to help that child, in whatever fashion was appropriate. But there wasn't this sense that somebody was responsible. The thing that fuels that fire are these highly publicized cases that come to trial, and in which there are huge awards for the family.

Most of the time when there are problems, it's not clear where the fault lies. In fact, most of the time, in Dr. Nichols's view, it is quite clear that the fault does not lie with the obstetrician. Yet, people see those $2,500,000 awards, and they get stirred into a frenzy. Especially when attorneys are out there advertising—IF YOU GET INTO AN ACCIDENT, CALL HAUGH & FOOTE! That sort of thing.

The upshot is that while Dr. Mark Nichols and his Pill Hill colleagues are glad they don't have to pay the malpractice-insurance premiums, it doesn't mean they don't think about the M-word all the time. They've even introduced training for the residents in what they call "risk management"—a catch-phrase for trying to prevent malpractice cases.

When you have a baby, anything can happen. Anything. He should know.

Dr. Nichols and his wife had a set of twins, delivered by cesarean section right down the hall from the office where he comes to work—Grant and Cameron, monozygotic—identical—twins who grew to maturity in the same sac. But they weren't really identical. Grant had massive *hydrocephalus,* "water on the brain." Here are two genetically identical babies; one has hydrocephalus, the other is normal. Maybe it's genetic, maybe it isn't. Is it some environmental thing? If so, then whatever environmental thing happened to one should happen to the other, right? But it didn't.

It was in August 1984. Dr. Nichols had just finished his residency the year before. He and his wife, Jan, a nurse-practitioner in pediatric cardiology, had waited to start their family until he was done training. She had come up with him from California, and they had lived together several years before marrying. There he was, a resident, and she was working in Pill Hill's pediatric intensive care, but they hardly ever got to see each other. When he was on call, he'd carve out twenty minutes to run over to South Hospital so they could eat their bag lunches together. She worked the evening shift, three to eleven, so when he wasn't on call, he'd come home and collapse into a heap, and she'd come home around eleven-thirty or twelve, wake him up, and they'd spend an hour together. An awful existence, reason aplenty to delay having kids.

She got pregnant, they bought Huggies, and then, with the very first ultrasound, at ten weeks, the Nicholses knew they had twins on the way. At eighteen weeks, they also knew that one baby was hydrocephalic, the other was not.

When they did another scan at eighteen weeks, Mark and Jan Nichols were looking at the ultrasound screen with the technician. Even though Jan hadn't seen that much obstetric scanning, as soon as the tech put the scanner on Grant's head, it was very clear he had hydrocephalus. They all looked at each other, not saying much. Jan could sense immediately that something was wrong, really bad. So Dr. Mark Nichols ended up making the diagnosis of hydrocephalus on his own son.

Ethically, it was one of the most difficult scenarios imaginable. Every three weeks, another scan, and oh God, it was worse *every time! every time! every time!* But a normal baby also was blissfully tucked into that warm, safe snuggery inside. They couldn't bring themselves to terminate the life of that baby along with the hopeless one's. Should they destroy the baby with the hydrocephalus or deliver it by cesarean, try to salvage it?

Gathering as much information as they could, they realized the child would most likely be "severely affected." But the information was shaky. While hydrocephalus has been around a long time, it is usually diagnosed late in pregnancy, when already severe, so there was little information about its impact throughout the pregnancy, or about the outcome for the baby. In hydrocephalus the ventricles fill with water, flattening the brain matter against the skull. Apparently, there was about a 20 percent chance he would be neurologically normal. An eight-in-ten chance there would be at least some degree of impairment. Maybe the damage would be minimal. Maybe not.

They didn't want everyone in the hospital to be in on it, talking about it. The ultrasound people were very careful to make sure that nobody was around when they came for the scans. The reason for all the secrecy was simple: The Nicholses were deciding whether to terminate one baby, and a lot of people in obstetrics and pediatrics would never consider that as an ethical option. It was the most difficult decision they had ever made, the right one for them, maybe not the right one for other people. Having made their decision, they didn't want to have to debate it or discuss it.

About a month before the scheduled cesarean section, they told people, selecting a few L&D nurses to assist in the surgery. They consulted Perinatalogist Dr. John Bissonnette. Jan's obstetrician was there, of course. From pediatrics they chose two faculty members to attend the delivery. While no heroics were to be done for their hydrocephalic baby, they wanted to ensure that if the normal infant was in any trouble, he would be well cared for. The couple met with all these people, told them what was likely to happen, what they wanted to have happen if things didn't work out as predicted.

By the day of the cesarean, the couple were basket cases. Jan had an epidural, and had been sedated. As planned, the hydrocephalic infant's head was drained before the first cut was made in Jan's abdomen. To the horrified surprise of all, he emerged vigorous, bright-eyed, looking around, emitting a loud squall. His "normal" brother, once taken from his mother's belly, proved to be weak, hypertensive, and in need of resuscitation. Gradually, he came around.

Jan Nichols could have delivered her twins anywhere in the city—in fact, she had originally planned to go to Good Sam—but the couple knew they needed the kind of care they would get on Pill Hill's 4NE. No other hospital in town would have been as accommodating.

The pediatricians seemed eager to have both babies taken home. Both were stable enough to leave the hospital, and their parents, the nurse-practitioner and doctor, were able to handle any medical problem that might come up. The hospital staff were supremely compassionate and caring, but it was also emotionally and ethically so difficult for everyone that it was a huge relief when Jan and Mark Nichols took their sons home.

Because of his hydrocephalus, Grant couldn't swallow, so he had to have a tube placed in his mouth and stomach. Grotesquely collapsed by its predelivery draining, his head soon reaccumulated fluid and was once again massive. Eventually, he was having so many seizures that he was put on phenobarbitol.

Four or five days after he went home, Grant Nichols died, aspirating his own vomit, a common way for hydrocephalic infants to die. He was three weeks old.

Cameron, Grant's twin brother, is now three and three-quarters years old. His little brother Alex is eight months old.

Dr. Mark Nichols, head of Pill Hill's OB/GYN residency program, has his heart in his work. Sometimes, though, the work fills up too many corners of his heart. Dearly, passionately, he wishes he could spend more time with his wife and their two little boys. With the two residents needing to be gone, though, he'll have to cover call with the rest of the department's faculty.

He'll be spending more time here, not less.

CHAPTER FOUR

("I don't like to think about my patients' pasts and futures," says the pregnant intern.)

As CHAIRMAN OF HIS department at Oregon Health Sciences University, Dr E. Paul Kirk is answerable for the works. His bailiwick includes the outpatient clinic, which treats private patients as well as women receiving public assistance, the training of the residents, and what actually happens on both floors of the hospital's maternity ward—the Labor and Delivery Department on 4NE, and the Mother-Baby Unit one floor down, on 3NW.

It is not a one-man show, of course, and in all of this, Dr. Kirk has good help.

One of the main functions of a teaching hospital is to train residents to be good specialists. An OB/GYN residency extends over four arduous years. The first-year residents are called "interns"; fourth-year residents are the "chiefs," chief residents. Typically, two hundred soon-to-graduate medical students from all over the country apply to do their OB/GYN residency at Oregon Health Sciences University.

Out of those ten-score applicants, seventy are interviewed. Only six are chosen. Pill Hill's OB/GYN residency program looks for the usual qualifications: top grades, community service, a commitment to the specialty, and glowing letters of recommendation.

When it comes down to it, however, the decision often turns on interpersonal skills, on how well the doctor-to-be is going to work with patients, how well he or she is going to empathize. "Team players" are consciously sought, people who are likely to support other residents in what is undeniably a stressful program. The selection system is weighted 60 percent on a candidate's *curriculum vitae*—the grades, med school dean's letter, and other recommendations—and the other 40 percent on the interview, wherein the prospect spends a half day at OHSU being eyed by three or four faculty members and a like number of current residents. The theory is that if you're going to have to work with someone day and night for four years, you might as well pick someone you can stand.

A first-year OB/GYN resident on Pill Hill spends much time on 4NE, seeing all of the patients who come in. A patient's history is taken, she is assessed, her treatment plan is developed, and she is closely monitored. A senior resident is consulted for anything out of the ordinary. Low-risk deliveries are performed, second- and third-year residents called in for the high-risk cases. As a new resident's skills increase, minor surgeries—episiotomy repairs, say—are done. Toward the end of that first year, the resident may assist at forceps deliveries, and participate in cesarean sections performed under the eagle eye of staff and senior residents. Time is spent in the outpatient clinic, following the pregnancies and other gynecological needs of patients.

All of this, for all residents throughout their four years, is accomplished during a nightmarish schedule of shifts. Every third or fourth night, there is a thirty-six-hour shift—say, work all day Sunday, from 7:00 or 8:00 A.M., through Sunday night, through all day Monday, then leave the hospital at 6:00 P.M. or so Monday night. Then sleep—heavy, exhaustion-drugged sleep—and back again at the hospital at 6:00 or 7:00 A.M. Tuesday. Then home Tuesday night at 6:00 or 7:00 P.M., back to work twelve hours later, at 6:00 A.M. Wednesday morning, to start another thirty-six-hour marathon.

The resident may spend those hours in the clinic, treating the usually pregnant outpatient women, then up on the labor and delivery floor all night, this under the best of circumstances, barring illness among the residents or family emergencies. An OB/GYN resident's work week lasts anywhere from seventy-two to one hundred or so hours. During call on L&D, first- and second-year residents are up all night. The senior residents—the third- and fourth-years—may, if it's a slow night, go to bed in one of the bare "call rooms" upstairs, to get three or four hours of sleep. There have been occasions when residents have fallen asleep in the middle of a cesarean section—lurching, in fact, straight toward the patient on the operating table. Miraculously, it seldom happens.

There is considerable controversy about the effects of sleep deprivation. Different residents seem to handle the lack of sleep during a day and a half differently. ("You wouldn't want your *mail* delivered by someone who's been up thirty-six hours, much less your baby!" one resident grumbles.) But the consensus seems to be that it's just one of those things, and you get used to it. What other choice is there?

Books and books have been written about the process of becoming a physician, and residency training is really *it,* the apprenticeship, the proving ground. At times, it even seems like hazing of young doctors: We had to go through it, now it's your turn. What keeps Dr. Mark Nichols coming back day after day, is the excitement of people starting their internship—and four years later, they're competent specialists.

But when an applicant comes for an interview, if even one interviewer, faculty or resident, says "No," then that's it—the application is not even considered. They go for "nice people" here, people who will add to the camaraderie and spirit. This program has a reputation for residents who really do care about each other. And that's the way it's going to stay.

Not that that's all there is to it. There has to be a touch of the surgeon's personality, an ability to make difficult decisions in a short period of time, to act quickly and effectively. In obstetric emergencies, you can't mealy-mouth around, when it's time to make a decision. At the same time you've got to balance this with a personality, an approach, a style that's almost the antithesis of that stereotypical surgeon personality. You've got to communicate well, spend the extra time to really reassure patients, be sympathetic to what—for the typical busy physician—might be a less significant complaint. All these factors go into building a strong relationship with patients.

The ideal resident would be someone with a touch of that surgeon personality, who can at the same time realize that there's a need to spend extra minutes with the patient, to address the psychosocial issues the patient is facing. More women are going into medicine, and in the past decade, not surprisingly, the specialty of obstetrics and gynecology has really started to attract more and more females. Sometimes, Dr. Nichols thinks a lot of women go into OB/GYN for political reasons, to be on the cutting edge of a feminist issue. Then they find themselves committed to a specialty with some special demands, yet turning back is hard because they've already devoted so much time to it. Here they are, getting close to the end of their reproductive careers, and they find themselves wanting to have a baby, wanting to have a marriage, wanting to complete their professional training, wanting to have a private life. But you can't have it all.

You cannot have it all.
Nobody can.

1530: 3:30 P.M.

A rainy April Tuesday, and all the rooms in the Labor and Delivery Department are filled. If anybody knows you can't have it all, it's First-Year Resident Tracey Delaplain, standing on sore feet at the nurses' station looking through the chart of Marie Henson, the woman laboring in Room 2. Marie is twenty-nine and this will be her third kid, after bearing twin boys three years ago. Seemed like a nice enough lady when Tracey took a look at her a few minutes ago. Tracey wonders what Marie's story is. Not that it matters, one way or the other.

Tracey Delaplain herself is pregnant, really pregnant, and if there's one place she doesn't want to have her baby, it's here on Pill Hill. Unless something goes wrong with the delivery, anyway. She wants to be pampered, have a nice room. Over at Good Sam, they have big rooms with lots of overstuffed chairs where your family can be with you the whole time. And stereos. She deserves it, by God.

There's nothing flashy about Tracey. She's always been steady and sensible, with a dry sense of humor. Even as a kid, she never dreamed of starring in the movies, or being a model. In grade school she was the one the teachers had pass out the thumbtacks, monitor the playground. When Tracey was . . . oh, fifteen or sixteen, she decided she wanted to be a doctor. She'd been talking about being a nurse ever since she was a little kid. Then a family friend, a doctor, talked to her, and when he found out she was interested in medicine itself, not just nursing per se, he talked Tracey into aiming for medical school instead. It was a pretty big dream for Tracey Lane of Carson City, Nevada, youngest of four. Her mother was a housewife. Her father had never finished high school, though he had worked his way up to an executive kind of position with a casino in nearby Reno.

They were all encouraging enough—like, "Oh, neat, Tracey wants to be a doctor!" But they kept talking about how were they—how was she—going to pay for it? Tracey did really well in school, going straight ahead, enrolling in a pre-med program at the University of Nevada. Just acting like it was all going to happen. Even though her family were pretty straight and Catholic, Tracey lived with her boyfriend, Tom, through college, and they got married their senior year. Then, sure enough, Tracey got into the state's med school in Reno. Even with all the scholarships and grants, together Tracey and Tom owe something like $50,000—and it'll be another two years before she's earning anything at all.

In July, when the baby comes, Tom will take a couple weeks off from his job, and Tracey will take eight weeks' maternity leave. Then it will be day care during the days, with Tom taking care of it (him? her?) at nights when Tracey's on one of her thirty-six-hour shifts. That's the plan, the best they can come up with. A baby wasn't exactly in the master plan, but they're pleased and excited about it now.

Every so often, especially when she's feeling tired and discouraged, Tracey has this nightmare that her kids will wake up one day and ask who the woman is who has dinner with

65

them once a week. She just hopes they don't say, "But that *other* lady is really nice!" She has lots of worries. One of the biggest ones is that the baby will love Tom more than her. Tom says that's not going to happen, that she'll have "quality time" together with the kid. But it's really hard.

Not that there haven't been hard choices all along, and a whole bunch just lying in wait. Tracey and Tom have given up their free time. There was no free time period, during medical school. Never money to travel or for extra, fun stuff during college and med school. Some of her friends, after high school a bunch of them went right out to work, and they had the fancy new cars and the fancy new clothes, you know. Pretty much the same as every college student puts up with—you see these guys you went to high school with having a great time while you're hitting books and working part time to supplement the scholarships and grants. On one level, you don't mind the sacrificing because you know where you're going. At the end of it all, you're a doctor. But when you go through eight years of it, it's really a drag.

And then there's Tom's sacrifices. Tracey made the choice to finish medical school and go *wherever* for residency, no matter what happened with their relationship. It's worked out fine. Even though he trained as a seismologist, Tom couldn't get a job in his field, so he's working with computers. He likes it, a lot. But you never know.

And the sleep—or rather, the lack of sleep! When she gets home, all Tracey wants to do is sleep. Tom understands. By now, he ought to. Once in a while, they get a chance to go out on the boat, and that's fun. Hang on, and we'll make it, Tracey and Tom take turns saying to each other. Sometimes, she doesn't cope very well. At the end of thirty-six hours of being awake, if you haven't had any sleep at all, you don't cope anymore. You're just too tired. She's gets impatient, more tearful, snaps at people, gets more frustrated with patients. That's the biggest thing to get over, the sleep deprivation. So when she leaves here, Tracey sleeps as much as she can, at the expense of everything else. Especially now that she's pregnant.

There are all kinds of studies showing how a medical residency and pregnancy don't mix too well. There's a higher frequency of prematurity, of lower birth weight, that kind of thing.

Probably, the stress isn't hurting Tracey's baby at all. Probably. But you never know.

1542: 3:42 P.M.

In Room 2 twenty-nine-year-old Marie Henson has been in labor for seven hours, since a little before nine this morning, her long blond hair damp and tangled. There she was, before her eyes were really open, just standing in the kitchen dumping nasty little sugar-coated, fluorescent-colored, animal-shaped bits of cereal into the bowls with the Raggedy Anns and Andys for her three-year-old twin sons, who won't eat anything but that vile stuff, when *whoosh!* out comes this hot splash from between her legs.

Naturally, life being what it is (which is to say predictable in these matters), Bill had just left for the plant. So Marie had to call her sister-in-law to come and get her and take her up to The Hill, and drop the boys off at Bill's mother's. She was at the hospital a good hour and a half before Bill could get up here.

But everything's okay now. Bill brought one of those Garfield balloons that says YOU'RE ONE OF A KIND! He is something, this guy. Even though the twins aren't his—they were just babies when Marie and Bill met, right after she had just gotten in and out of the world's quickest-and-worst marriage and divorce—Bill treated them right off like they were his own sons.

When they were courting, and the babies just a few months old, sometimes they'd tuck them in for the night right there in the bathtub of Bill's apartment over on Northwest Overton! He'd change their dirty diapers, even. But he says he would like just one more kid. A girl, if she wouldn't mind.

Three kids are plenty, too, for Marybeth O'Grady. Last night, in the same room where Marie Henson now labors, Marybeth's 9½-pound son debuted with the help of Mityvac suction, First-Year Resident Gary Hoffman and the moral support of freckled, red-haired father Dennis. In fact, given the financial state of the O'Grady household—which includes Marybeth and Dennis, seven-year-old Patrick and Molly, four, and Marybeth's mother—when you get right down to it, *two* kids would have been just fine. But Joshua Matthew is a good kid. Marybeth can tell that already. And *sooooooooo* cute. The image of his father.

The lights are glaring in OR2, where Marybeth is being prepped for her tubal ligation.

"He was so *cute*," says a green scrubs-suited nurse, who was there when the child was born last night.

Marybeth grins her huge smile at this.

"He was so *big*," she replies, laughing.

In the scrub room between the two operating rooms, Residents Elizabeth Newhall and Brenda Kehoe prepare themselves for Marybeth's surgery. Liz Newhall's lush red hair is pulled back, secured to the nape of her neck with a red rubber band, and covered completely by a blue paper snood that looks like an old-fashioned plastic shower cap.

The surgical scrub is a time-honored procedure, with its own formal choreography. Standing at opposite sinks in the small room, controlling the water's flow with foot pedals, the two women first wash their hands and arms with a soap solution, removing obvious dirt and oil. Then they open small packets with sponges impregnated with an iodine solution. Arms lifted up, hands bent with fingers tipped up, they scrub vigorously—the palms, the nails, down to the elbows. After five minutes, they rinse, and all the sudsy, contaminated water, tinted orange from the iodine, runs off at the elbows.

It is generally considered that the scrub should be a thorough five minutes, and though some hold to the belief that the day's first scrub should take ten minutes, with less time spent on subsequent scrubs through the day. Since Marybeth's tubal ligation is elective, no emergency, there is time to do a thorough scrub. Were she lying on the operating table awaiting a crash—emergency—cesarean section, the overriding issue would not be possible contamination but rather to get a dying baby out. In that case, both surgeons and patient would do a "splash prep."

Arms raised in front, above waist level, without touching the connecting door, Residents Brenda Kehoe and Liz Newhall amble into OR2. A scrub tech—in this case, a medical student—hands them each a sterile towel to dry their still-wet hands. Half a towel is used to dry the right hand, the other half dries the left. A sterile, disposable gown is carefully draped over each resident, the hands and arms carefully kept from touching anything but the gown's sleeves. Then the scrub tech sterilely gloves each doctor in turn. Often—usually, for some doctors—a second pair of sterile latex gloves is put on as an extra precaution against direct contact with a patient's possibly HIV-contaminated blood and other bodily fluids.

"How're you doing?" asks Liz Newhall, voice filtering through her blue paper mask.

"I'm nervous," says the now-slender blonde stretched out on the operating table. "I'm nervous about having my tubes tied. These operations, they don't always work, do they? I have a friend, and . . . well, her cousin. . . . " Her voice trails off.

"I wouldn't worry," replies Liz Newhall. "It's only once in every four hundred times that the operation doesn't prove effective."

"Great," says Marybeth O'Grady. "And what are you supposed to do with that every-four-hundred-times baby?" The three women laugh at the weak, nervous joke.

Dr. Betsy Soifer doesn't laugh. Above her green scrubs with their pink drawstring waistband, the staff anesthesiologist wears clear-framed glasses, glittery square metal earrings, a blue jacket, and a round green button that reads: TRAUMA. ASK ME ABOUT MY ROLE.

A few feet from the door into OR2, OB/GYN Department Chairman E. Paul Kirk sits behind the counter of the nurses' station, talking into the phone. It seems that another Portland hospital wants to send over a laboring woman. Not, as it turns out, because she is at risk for complications. Not because they don't have room for her. No, the hospital down the hill and across town wants Pill Hill to take this woman off its hands because, quite simply, she is nonpaying. While not on welfare, she is one of the medically indigent.

Dr. Kirk is very angry. All his labor rooms are full, and there are women downstairs in the Mother-Baby Unit who will need to come up soon.

"If she comes here, we'll have to put her in a bed in the hall!"

He listens to the response.

"Tell me this," he asks. "Do you know the figures of our patients here, over a year's time, who *we* care for with no reimbursement?"

The chairman listens.

"I think you are confusing the issue," he replies, speaking slowly and distinctly, as though to a very young child. "We are not talking about '*the system.*' We are talking about *space!*"

Again, he listens to the hospital on the other end of the line.

"No," says Dr. Kirk, "you are *not* guaranteed payment. But there's nothing that says you *can't* take care of her!"

Again, the other hospital responds, and the chairman sighs.

"If she *comes,* we'll take care of her, yes. Yes."

Dr. Kirk hangs up the phone.

1640: 4:40 P.M.

Down in the Mother-Baby Unit, LaTonya Jordan in Room 11 gazes incuriously at her new baby daughter, fussing in the bassinet alongside her bed. She was born at 11:15 last night. LaTonya is sore, and she is feeling very cranky. She informs a nurse that she is *not* thirteen years old. She turned fourteen last month. The *beginning* of last month.

One of the reasons LaTonya is so bummed out is that that Marcus, who got her pregnant, hasn't come to see her and the baby yet. He's seventeen, and goes to Vocational Village, an alternative high school for dropouts run by the Portland School District. Just wait till that fool Marcus tries to get some more pussy off of her, he'll see! Lying there in the narrow, white-sheeted bed, LaTonya tries to fold her arms across her chest, but it doesn't work. Her milk is coming in, and her huge breasts are tender.

70

Shit. Nobody told her about this.

Across the room lies a wan brunette, her stomach only slightly distended with the baby the doctors are trying to keep inside for at least three more weeks. She stares listlessly at Phil Donahue on the TV screen above, where people are shouting about sex education for the mentally retarded.

"How come *she* gets to have that thing to change the station?" LaTonya whines to the nurse. "It's *my* turn, ain't it?"

The nurse tilts her head questioningly toward the thin young woman in the other bed, who shrugs and shakes her head with a small, tired smile. The remote control is transferred to LaTonya, who makes a snort of triumph as she zaps the set.

On Channel 2, Oprah Winfrey is interviewing women, onstage and in the worked-up audience, about something called "fatal attractions."

1734: 5:34 P.M.

In MBU's Room 12, across the hall from LaTonya, Cammie Edwards, whose son was born in the ambulance yesterday, is still sleeping off her drugs of the past few days. Her long red silky tresses are spread out across the pillow, one thin freckled arm raised up and around her head. Stretched out, asleep on the bed with Cammie, is her scruffy boyfriend, his arm under her neck and around her fragile shoulders.

In slumber, the pair look like small, frail children, perhaps ten years old. Whacked-out Gretel with her Hansel, sleeping in the forest beneath a tree, in their dreams momentarily sheltered from the Wicked Witch hell-bent on their destruction.

Hilary Blanchard, holed up in her room in the Mother-Baby Unit, wishes it were possible to take a quiet nap in this dump. She closes her eyes and does some deep breathing. (*Long, slow, deep exhalation . . . take in strength and energy. Long, slow, comfortable exhalation . . . release the stress, let it go.*) Surprise, surprise, it doesn't work. From the depths of her mind, Hilary slides out one of her favorite memories, playing it on what she thinks of as her own private inside-her-head movie screen.

71

One Monday afternoon after school, back when Hilary Blanchard was a six-year-old named Hilary Grey, living with her parents and younger brother in a nice apartment overlooking Central Park West, she went with her mother on their weekly "Mommy Adventure Day" to a very old, old building in a park in Upper Manhattan. This, the art historian told her first grader, was called The Cloisters. As was her habit, Hilary diddled and dawdled her way through the museum, wondering how long they had to stay before she'd get her ice cream cone. And then she saw it.

The little girl in long blond pigtails stood still and transfixed. Clad in her private-school uniform (blue and green plaid skirt, tomato soup-besmottered white blouse, navy cardigan, one navy knee-high drooping down around one skinny ankle, the other inexplicably staying up around the bony knee, brown Oxfords hopelessly scuffed), she was gone. Hilary's mother, mystified and slightly amused by her odd child, explained that what they were looking at was called a *tapestry*. And she told her what she knew about it.

The animal is only pretend, Hilary's mother told her, and it's called a *unicorn*. Its body is like a horse—isn't it?—but you'll notice that it has a big horn growing out of its forehead. It has a little beard like a goat's. And its tail is like a lion's—see! There are seven tapestries to tell the story. The others show how the unicorn is chased and captured by the men, and how they kill it. But look—you see that the unicorn comes back to life. And then, at the end of the story, the poor unicorn is being held captive, tied to the tree inside the round wooden fence.

Who made it? asked the child. Is it very old? Why is it here? Can we take it home with us, and put it on the wall in my room?

Hilary's mother explained that the tapestry was woven more than five centuries ago—that's five hundred years!—for a rich and powerful man in France. The grave-faced child heard from her mother that day that the fenced-in unicorn once hung in the sleeping quarters of a great nobleman, who probably rolled it up with the other six hangings, carrying them by horseback whenever he traveled. That way, he would feel cozy and at home, no matter where he went.

The tapestries stayed in the same family, hanging on the walls of their great castle, called a *chateau,* until the French Revolution. Then they were stolen by angry peasants, along with other things from the chateau. A lot of beautiful things were broken up and ruined. But sixty years later, a man in the family that owned the chateau searched all over the countryside, trying to find his family's treasures. And what do you know! He found these tapestries—these beautiful cloth pictures telling the story of the unicorn—covering up a bunch of dirty vegetables inside somebody's barn out in the country! So he just had them mended, and put them back on the castle walls, where they had been for so many hundreds of years.

Hilary was fascinated. Her mother told her how the unicorns came across the ocean, to an art gallery in this very city, and then they were bought by a man named John D. Rockefeller.

"Like the skating-rink Rockefeller?" the child asked.

"The very one," her mother answered. "And then Mr. Skating-Rink Rockefeller gave the unicorns to the Metropolitan Museum of Art—where they have the Egyptian mummies that you like—and the museum put them in this place with other old, old things."

The next day, when Hilary got home from school, she found a print of "The Unicorn in Captivity" on her bedroom wall, framed and matted with the same rosy-peach color of the flowers in the wallpaper. It presented a strange contrast (over the years, often commented upon by her parents' friends) to the Barbie dolls and the stuffed animals. Like the French counts, she kept her fenced-in unicorn there on the wall opposite her bed, to gaze upon before falling asleep.

In later years, studying art history, Hilary would come to grasp the powerful Christian iconography of the tapestries, how each of the dozens of *millefleurs,* the woven flowers, added allegorical richness to the symbolism understood, once upon a time, by the weavers and other people who beheld the unicorn's progress on the chateau walls.

Yet, it was always the sweet, sad expression on the unicorn's face that enchanted, that soothed and comforted first the little girl, and then the young woman. The framed print went with Hilary to college in California, and from there to

73

graduate school in Massachusetts, and to her new home in Central Oregon. And now, here.

When Hilary's mother arrived last night from New York, she presented her daughter with a huge needlepoint canvas, a meticulously painted copy of "The Unicorn in Captivity," ready to be stitched.

"Where on earth did you *find* this?" asked the daughter.

"Find it? I painted it for you to work on while you're here," answered the mother. "I suspected you might enjoy the company of an old friend. And I'm going to teach you how to do petit point."

Hilary turned her face away so that her mother couldn't see the tears starting.

"Oh, for heaven's sake, Hilary, don't cry—you'll just get me going! Sooner or later, this will all be over!"

Resident Karen Hill comes into Lily Pratt's room in the Mother-Baby Unit across the hall from Hilary Blanchard.

"How're you feeling, Mrs. Pratt?" asks the doctor.

"Oh, fine," replies Lily. "But you know what's bugging me?"

"What?"

"Well, my older sister's having her twenty-fifth anniversary today, and the celebration's Saturday. And I hate to ruin that! But then, I was talking to my husband, and he said just forget about the anniversary and just concentrate on *this*! But I know that they'll worry, that's the thing. Are you sure we have to start the labor?"

(Secretly, silently, Lily wonders if they're going to induce her labor because she's so overweight. She is ashamed to ask this.)

"There's nothing the matter with your pregnancy, or with your baby," replies the resident, sitting down on the chair alongside Lily's bed. "Everything's developed at this stage. We're just going to keep you at bedrest until your cervix is favorable enough to be delivered. That's kind of the plan."

"Why isn't it favorable?" asks Lily.

"Well, it's kind of rock-hard," replies Karen Hill. "And before labor, it has to soften up. It has to dilate some, and move into a good position. Yours is not acting like it wants to go into labor yet. And if we try when your cervix is like a rock, it just doesn't work. So we'd like it to change a little bit, okay?"

Lily nods, though she doesn't really understand all this.

"But I think you're stable, and your blood pressure's great. As long as the baby's okay, we can hold off."

Patting Lily's bare left arm (large, soft, and freckled), Dr. Karen Hill leaves the room to begin her long trek back upstairs to L&D.

Up in L&D, First-Year Resident Tracey Delaplain, who delivered Cammie Edwards's afterbirth, remembers that the young redhead didn't even know she'd delivered her son in the ambulance yesterday afternoon, didn't even need an episiotomy repair. Tracey doesn't like to think about her patients' pasts or futures. It makes it too hard.

After all this time, through medical school back in Reno, and after all these months of residency, it still astounds Tracey that so many women who come in here have *no* idea how pregnant they are, or when they got pregnant, or what their periods are. And they're not the least bit upset about the fact that their membranes ruptured two days ago, and that they might be having a premature baby. They just don't understand what that means. It's frustrating.

And this afternoon Tracey especially doesn't like the directive she's been given about Melody Richards, the eighteen-year-old blonde who's been huffing and puffing away in Room 8 since a little after five this morning. Melody is not supposed to hold—or even *see*—her baby once it arrives. The kid is supposed to be whisked off to the INCU across the hall as soon as it emerges. And while other mothers are cooing over their newborns down in the Mother-Baby Unit, Melody will instead be transported, postpartum, all the way over to South Hospital.

This complicated set of orders, devised to "make things easier" for Melody, to prevent her "bonding" with her baby, has been transmitted by Rebekah, mother of seven and a fellow member of the Mormon church. She has been keeping an eye on Melody for three months now, ever since she arrived in Portland from Utah.

Melody figures she's been in twelve foster homes since

she was nine. That's when her mom, who'd been in and out of mental hospitals since long before Melody was even born, decided to let the state of Utah take all six kids off her hands and stick them into foster homes.

For a couple of years there in the foster homes, heartsick and missing her mother and her brothers and sisters, Melody tried to keep her head down and mind her own business, to stay out of trouble. Lot of good that did. In the first place, right off, the two older sons of the foster mother did stuff to her while one of the other foster kids, a big fat girl named Trixie, held her down. When Melody told her social worker about it, they just moved her into another home, where the mother was drunk all the time and didn't even get the kids up for school in the morning, and there wasn't ever anything to eat. The third place—or was it the fourth?—they were Mormons, and that's where Melody joined the Church, and the family was real nice, but then the father got transferred to another state, and Melody was put in another awful place, and that's when she got good at running away.

One of the really crummy parts in all this was that Melody would see her real mother every few months, and she'd tell her about the stuff that was happening. Only her mother never did believe her, and she'd always tell Melody and the other kids that they were going to get back together like a real family soon, like next month. Only it would never happen, you know?

Melody was out on her own for a couple of years when she got pregnant by this guy who had just broken up with his girlfriend, and when Melody told him about the baby, he said it wasn't his probably, and anyway he was thinking of going back to his *real* girlfriend and that was the last she saw of him. And when she told her mother about it, and that she had gone back to the Church and that the Church was finding a nice family to raise the baby, her mother laid this big fat guilt trip on her about how she better keep the baby, because family's family.

And Melody, as mad as she got, couldn't see any sense to saying to her mother how that family's family stuff was a big fat joke, seeing as it was coming from her.

Everything has been arranged, every small detail, for the instant adoption of Melody's baby by a Mormon couple who,

76

as the blond teenager shudders her way through labor, are packing their bags in Provo, ready to catch the 11:50 P.M. train out of Salt Lake City. The bishop of Melody's church helped her choose the family. He gave her a choice, provided a trio of couples for Melody to eenie-meenie-miney-mo from: their hobbies, professions, what kind of home they have. (Though nothing she could really, you know, identify them from. It's better that way, she knows, even though Melody sure would like to see a picture of them.)

This couple has already spent so much money on their new house with the nursery all decorated with teddy bears. (They're *real* partial to teddy bears, Rebekah tells Melody, over and over and over. Isn't that *sweet*?) They've spent so much money on all this, and that's how come they can only afford to take the train, not an airplane, to Portland to pick up the baby.

But not to worry. They'll have plenty of new clothes and diapers and everything ready to take the baby with them. And she does understand—doesn't she?—why it's best not to look at the baby and hold it?

"Melody is the most *selfless* person I know," Rebekah croons repeatedly, pacing Room 8, seldom looking away from Melody's face.

"She knows she's doing what's *best*!"

1907: 7:07 P.M.

According to a clipping from *The Oregonian,* pinned to the cork board on the wall between OR2 and the coffee/supply room, the most popular name for baby girls in Oregon this year is Ashley.

Right now, in Room 2 in the Labor and Delivery Department of Oregon Health Sciences University, one small girl named Ashley Marie Henson is making her laborious way into the world. Her parents, Bill and Marie Henson, can't wait to see her. The still-cheerful Marie writhes and grunts with the effort, insisting between the powerful contractions that this is a piece of cake compared to giving birth to twin sons. Also in the room are little Ashley's aunt Marge, Nurse-Midwife Linda

Lutz, two nurse-midwifery students, and a medical student whose ID photo makes him look a lot more like a young Robert Redford than he really does.

If Marie Henson thinks it's hard work getting her daughter out (and it is) she should try being the baby. All these months of sweet, sloshing warmth, followed by a torturous trip down the birth canal. And then out: into a shock of cool air and sharp noise. It's enough to make anybody cry.

Ashley Marie Henson, having her umbilical cord cut by her father, lets out a howl of dismay.

"*Beautiful* work!" This, from Nurse-Midwife Linda Lutz.

"I gotta call some people that'll be mad if I don't. Jack and Connie. And Larry and Lisa!" This, from Bill, the new father.

"Don't forget your mom. And my stepmom!" This, from Marie, who holds her little girl, stroking one soft rose cheek with the back of her right index finger.

2015: 8:15 P.M.

This is Zanna Morrison's first baby, and so far the so-called glorious birthing process has been a real bitch. She's been in labor for almost four days—in the hospital since Saturday night. Her boyfriend, Shawn, has been a champ, though for a while there this afternoon, when they were putting that cone thing on the baby's head, sticking it up there through her vagina, he looked like he was about to barf.

The pretty doctor named Dr. Kennedy has been telling Zanna and Shawn that they might have to do a cesarean section, but they're not sure. That's pretty scary, but they keep telling Zanna it isn't her fault, that she didn't do anything wrong. It's because, maybe, the baby's cord could be wrapped around its neck, making it hard for it to get oxygen.

Chief Resident Kathy Kennedy has finally decided to section Zanna, whose labor has been dysfunctional all along. She has made no progress whatsoever in the past three hours. There have been big variable decelerations in the baby's heart rate. Dr. Kennedy thought it might all smooth out if they gave her a little Pitocin, but no dice. She had a fetal scalp pH test done with the cone, and indications are that the baby's blood oxygen level is low.

Dr. Kennedy enters Room 10. Zanna, exhausted, is leaning back into her pillow, and her boyfriend is stroking damp strands of long, dark hair from her forehead.

"We've decided that doing a cesarean section is best for the baby," Dr. Kennedy tells the young couple.

"Oh, *no!*" moans Zanna, beginning to cry.

"It'll be all right. Really it will," says Dr. Kennedy. Turning to the young father-to-be before she leaves the room, the resident tells Shawn that he can be there. If he wants to. And that a nurse will bring him a costume to put on for the operating room.

Exiting, Kathy Kennedy shuts the door quietly.

"Don't cry," says Shawn, stroking Zanna's cheek. "Don't cry. You heard the doctor. Everything's going to be okay." That's the way they've always been together: intense, dark-haired Zanna always the worrier, blond, curly-locked Shawn the cheerful optimist.

"Oh, come on, Shawn," Zanna snaps angrily. "Give me a break! They're going to cut my guts open! What if they miss and cut the baby?" She is crying harder now.

"Zanna!" Shawn is shocked. "They wouldn't want to do a cesarean section unless they have to. And I'll be there the whole time. I'll make sure they don't hurt you! Or the baby!" The couple clings to one another, rocking awkwardly, familiarly.

Zanna met Shawn when he came into the North Portland drugstore owned by her grandparents. She was working there on weekends, helping them out. Since she started school, Zanna had lived mostly with Gram and Gramps. After Zanna's father was killed in a motorcycle crash, her mom kept getting married and divorced, married and divorced. (What was she up to now—five? Six? It gets pretty hard to keep track of.) That Saturday, Shawn came in for some Gillette Foamy. Funny how you remember dumb little things like that. He looked a little familiar, and they got to talking, and discovered they both went to Roosevelt High, Zanna a junior and Shawn a sophomore. Zanna being so shy and all, and Shawn so outgoing, it was funny how well they got along right off. And

Gram and Gramps liked him right off, too, gave him a job weekends, and weren't all that surprised when they came home one night after Friday square dance club to catch the two of them on the living room sofa.

The biggest surprise of all turned out to be what happened next. Zanna's grandparents suggested that Shawn move in with them, and that they both finish up with high school. Then, if they still loved each other (and oh, they knew they would!), they could have a wedding with all the trimmings. Shawn's parents couldn't care less, just sort of shrugged when he told them of the plan. ("Do what you want," his mom said. "It's your life." Not that she didn't like Zanna, she was just like that.) Last August, after Shawn graduated, they almost got married, but then they discovered that Zanna was expecting, and she was damned if she was going to be a pregnant bride. Shawn thought that was kind of dumb, but he left it up to her.

"I love you so much, Zanna," he is saying now. "We are going to have the most beautiful baby in the world."

2025: 8:25 P.M.

Melody Richards is taking a walk in the hallway, her fresh young face contorted with the effort as she lumbers along, trying to hasten her labor. Her sister, holding Melody's elbow, moves along with her while the two pace slowly, back and forth, back and forth, along the corridor outside the labor and delivery rooms. A few feet away, talking on a wall phone, the vigilant Rebekah watches every step the teenager takes.

CHAPTER FIVE

Blood!

MOST OF US HAVE this thing about blood. Whenever we see it, a light flashes on somewhere in the brain: *Red Alert! Red Alert! Trouble! Someone's hurt! Someone's bleeding! Someone's dying, maybe even dead!* Many a medical student, in fact, makes a prompt and decisive shift in planned specialty on seeing— really seeing—blood up close. The crimson liquid splashes, oozes, gushes, issuing forth from the slice of scalpel, decorating in hues brilliant and ghastly the auto crash victim, brightly festooning the squirming, sticky body of the newborn child. ("Dermatology," thinks the blood-shy student. "Or ophthalmology. Psychiatry, maybe.")

One of medicine's blood sports, obstetrics and gynecology is not for the faint of heart. Six liters—ten to twelve pints— of blood course through the veins of the average female human being. The plasma carries food waste, the erythrocytes transport oxygen, and the leucocytes help to protect the baby against disease and infection. By about ten weeks into a normal pregnancy, the mother's plasma volume begins to increase until it plateaus at thirty to thirty-four weeks. At that point, the mean increase in plasma volume is 50 percent, although increases from 20 percent to 100 percent have been observed in normal pregnancies.

The mother's vastly increased blood volume protects her from possible hemorrhage at the time of delivery. Further, the increased volume of plasma helps dissipate fetal heat production, as well as provide increased renal filtration. And all those new red blood cells increase oxygen transport, meeting the needs of the child within.

There is plenty of blood to spare. Delivering a term infant vaginally usually results in a loss of about half a liter of blood; an uncomplicated cesarean section uses up about a liter. Normally, most of the blood loss associated with giving birth occurs within the first hour, with only about 80 milliliters lost over the next three days.

2028: 8:28 P.M.

Zanna Morrison has been moved down the hall, onto the table in the center of OR2, to be prepped for her cesarean section. Wearing a pink hospital gown that opens in the back, she nearly fills the table as Nurse Jennifer Ostermeyer helps her stretch out.

Zanna is shuddering through another contraction, a violent one this time, and moans as the nurse covers her with a sheet.

"Is this going to really hurt?" Zanna asks.

"No," Jennifer replies. "Once the anesthetic takes effect, you'll be completely numb, at least from the breasts on down."

"I don't want to see what they're doing," says Zanna. "All that blood and everything. Yuck."

"You won't," the nurse assures her. "When they're ready to go, they hang a sheet between your head and the rest of it."

"When does Shawn get to come in here?"

"Once they've put in the epidural. Half an hour or so. Don't worry, he'll be right here with you through the whole thing."

"Oh, good," says Zanna. "That's going to make it a lot better."

Through all this preliminary business, Staff Anesthesiologist Betsy Soifer and Resident Jeff Jones have been working at the head of the table, arranging Zanna's intravenous saline solution. Dr. Soifer puts a blood pressure cuff around Zanna's right arm.

"Now, this is going to feel tight in just a sec," she warns.

Dr. Jones puts a needle into the back of Zanna's left hand, and starts a drip of Lactated Ringer's, a saline solution that will continue to enter the patient's bloodstream throughout the surgery.

Dr. Soifer asks Zanna to roll onto her left side.

"I believe in telling patients exactly what's going on. No surprises," says the anesthesiologist.

"Oh, good," says Zanna.

"And now, the next stage is going to be—*tah-dah!*—the Cold Wet Back Stage."

As Dr. Soifer says this, the resident takes a small sponge attached to a six-inch-long white plastic handle and smears Betadine, a deep orange-hued antiseptic solution, onto a twelve-inch-wide circle on Zanna's back. The center, where the needle will go in, is swabbed with sterile alcohol-soaked gauze pads. Into the Betadine bull's-eye, to numb the area for the next step, he injects lidocaine, a local anesthetic.

The needle retracted, a tiny ruby of blood forms, growing larger until, finally, it runs in a small, neat stream down Zanna's back, reaching the orange border of Betadine.

"Okay, now," says Dr. Betsy Soifer. "I want you to arch your back like a mad, mad pussycat!"

Tears in her eyes, the patient obeys the doctor.

Carefully, carefully, a needle is inserted deep into Zanna's spine. She shrieks.

"Sorry," says Dr. Soifer. "Where did you feel that?"

"Right on my *butt*!"

Then follows an ornate procedure as the spinal anesthetic, a concoction of Marcaine with a little morphine, is injected into Zanna Morrison's spine. A type of plug is put in, with a thin wire threaded through. Finally, the procedure is completed, and Zanna is told to roll onto her back once again.

Nurse Jennifer rolls a Doppler, a device the size of a small cassette recorder, over Zanna's belly to listen one final time to the baby's heart rate. She has Zanna spread her knees apart and bring her feet together to create a small work area on the table for the next procedure. Gently spreading the lips of the young woman's vulva, Jennifer threads a clear plastic tube up through Zanna's urethra and into her bladder. Immediately, urine seeps through the plastic and into a bag, which will be replaced periodically over the next two or three days. The catheter will eliminate—along with the urine—the need for trips to the toilet to pee.

Finally, Jennifer wraps a wide, white elastic belt across Zanna's now-numb legs to keep them from flopping off the operating table.

"Can you feel this? This? This?" asks Dr. Jeff Jones, poking a short metal rod into Zanna's waist, moving it up her right side.

"*Now* I can," she says when the rod has reached her armpit. The rod-poking test shows comparable numbness on the patient's left side.

"Good," says Dr. Betsy Soifer. "Everything's just the way it's supposed to be. You're doing great, honey. Just great."

Like a charwoman on hands and knees scouring the kitchen linoleum, a nurse scrubs the lurid orange Betadine from side to side on Zanna's belly, all the way from her crotch to about six inches above her protuberant navel. The antiseptic transforms her glossy dark brown pubic hair to a ghastly, phosphorescent khaki green.

Emerging from the scrub room are Dr. Mark Nichols, Chief Resident Kathy Kennedy, and Residents Karen Hill and Bob Hicks. Through the hall doorway, from INCU down the hall, a pediatrics team sets up a warmer and equipment for the baby, who may be in distress once fetched from Zanna's belly.

A green cotton cloth serves as a curtain between the patient's head and the action that will take place at the site of her Betadined belly. A resident spreads out a large sterile drape with a strategic hole in the center with a transparent, adhesive surround that sticks to the outer edge of the patient's belly. The teenaged Shawn, clad in a blue jumpsuit worthy of the Starship *Enterprise,* is at the head of the table, behind the curtain with the frightened-looking Zanna's nonnumb head.

The overhead lamps are adjusted. Dr. Mark Nichols stands slightly back, on Zanna's left with Chief Resident Kathy Kennedy, poised to supervise Residents Bob Hicks and Karen Hill, who will be performing the surgery.

Finally, Third-Year Resident Bob Hicks, scalpel held steady, makes a low transverse cut about six inches along Zanna's satiny orange skin, an inch or so above the khaki-green pubic hair. Blood oozes up from the smile-shaped incision. Taking a lap sponge—a large white square of gauze—Second-Year Resident Karen Hill mops up the crimson fluid, revealing the subcutaneous yellow fatty layer.

With a sure hand, Dr. Hicks scalpels through this layer, which looks like the fat on a chicken being prepared for Sunday dinner. He cuts down to the fibrous layer sheathing her muscles—the fascial layer—and opens it sharply with a knife. The fascia is picked up with forceps and, with Mayo scissors, cut in a line similar to the skin incision. This releases the muscles from their confining sheath, allowing greater access into Zanna's belly. Kocher clamps are placed on the upper fascial edges for traction, and the fascia is cut away from the muscles of the anterior abdominal wall in the direction of Zanna's belly button. Dr. Hicks replaces the clamps on the lower edges of the fascia, and Dr. Karen Hill cuts the fascia away from the lower abdominal muscles, all the way to where they insert into Zanna's pubic bone.

The rectus muscles running up and down the length of Zanna's pregnant abdomen are separated bluntly by Dr. Hicks, and the thin peritoneal lining of the abdominal cavity is identified. A large pulling instrument called a Richardson retractor is placed in the incision, revealing blood and the blue-red gravid uterus. The peritoneum is opened high, away from Zanna's bladder, itself carried high into the abdominal cavity by her stretched and now-bloated uterus. Dr. Hicks picks up the peritoneum covering the uterus and, using Metzenbaum scissors, makes a transverse cut in the filmy lining.

The "bladder flap" thus created is now separated still further from the uterus, and it is pulled toward the pubic bone by Dr. Hill, who uses a second retractor called a "bladder blade." At this point, the bladder is pulled away, to keep it safe from potential harm by the uterine incision to come. The chore of positioning the bladder blade is handed off to scrub tech Dave Magilke.

The uterine "field" fully exposed, the bladder having been safely taken down from the lower uterine segment— now widely dilated with Zanna's infant's head—Dr. Hicks uses the scalpel again, making an incision in the lower uterine segment, a transverse cut with a slightly elliptical direction. He hooks his fingers, ghostly white in their double layer of latex gloves, into the angles of the wound, trying to pull it apart to split the circular myometrial muscles of the lower uterine segment. Tough and resistant, the muscles refuse to split manually.

"Use the scissors," Chief Resident Kathy Kennedy instructs the lower-level residents.

With Dr. Hill pulling hard on the Richardson retractor, the margins of the uterus are revealed. The dangerously pulsating uterine arteries can be palpated near the edges where the incision must be extended. The large, thin, blue dilated veins of the uterine plexus can also be seen—also perilously close to the margins of the impending incision.

As the uterus is opened, the amniotic sac—the "bag of waters"—wells up into the field of the incision. Parts of Zanna's baby can be seen beneath the bright sheen of the membranous sac. Glowing, pulsating from inside the young woman's abdomen, blood has been mopped up during the surgery with small gauze pads, the "sponges" that will be meticulously counted postsurgery.

Slick, beautiful, vivid, the blood has also been noisily slurped away throughout the operation by a device like the one dentists use to suck away saliva. A brilliant crimson scrim through which the drama is viewed, Zanna's blood imparts its regal sheen and beauty, its *realness,* to the proceedings.

I am Blood! I am Life!

With an instrument called an Allis clamp, Dr. Hicks makes a short, quick stabbing gesture toward the bag of waters. Gushes of amniotic fluid and blood splash forth from Zanna's belly, branding everyone within a two-foot radius of the birthing woman. Everyone laughs: residents, staff doctor, nurses, scrub technician.

Silence and urgency descend again as Dr. Hicks probes

with gloved hand, plunging through the elaborate wrappings, into the gift box, clear to the bottommost depths of the gaping wound. At last, a head is found and brought forth. It is a boy child, wearing a snug wrap of umbilical cord around his neck.

"*Aha!*" says Chief Resident Kathy Kennedy. "*That* explains his distress!"

In ritual swift and solemn, Dr. Hicks unwraps the slippery cord from the neck of the infant, while Dr. Hill suctions the baby's throat. These actions are met with loud indignant gasps from the child. The umbilicus is clamped, the cord severed. This is a whole person now, a creature able to live apart from his mother. Taking his first breath of the air on Planet Earth, the small boy bellows furiously, breaking the tension in OR2.

"Hel-*loooo!*" says a masked nurse, greeting the new child.

"Welcome!" says a doctor.

"Happy birthday, sweetheart!" chimes in another nurse from behind her mask.

"How big is he?" asks Dr. Kennedy, grinning behind her paper face mask. "I like it when they scream!"

Immediately, the little boy is handed to Pediatrics Resident Don Buffkin, who first runs his gloved hands over the newborn's form, cleaning him then with the heated flannel blankets. He finds a deep purple mark, shaped like the state of Texas.

"Hmmmm . . . ," the pediatrician says softly. "Looks like a little hemangioma here. Or a birthmark." Shawn, tears running into his paper mask, cranes his head in alarm from his girlfriend's face toward the baby.

"Don't worry!" says Dr. Buffkin. "People will only know that when they've been *really* friendly! Only his *close* friends will know!"

Relieved, the nineteen-year-old turns back to Zanna.

"He's beautiful," says Shawn to Zanna, his voice a half-sob.

"*Is* he?" she asks through her tears. "*Is* he?" Eyes shining, hands trembling, he strokes back her long, dark hair.

"Yes," he says, leaning forward to kiss her damp brow. "Oh, yes!"

The door to OR2 is open, the operating room silent but for the sound of hospital aide Filipinas Mugas Cox swabbing down the operating table with her bucket of disinfectant solution. The small woman wears the blue scrubs, long, dark tresses done up and hidden by the blue paper cover, meticulously made-up face obscured by the paper mask covering her nose and mouth. Blue paper booties cover her white shoes. Finishing the table, she begins cleaning the floor, the mop swiftly removing the traces of blood and amniotic fluid from Zanna Morrison's cesarean section, cleaning up the footprints made by bootie-covered shoes of the doctors, nurses and students in the operating room only a few minutes ago.

Alone at the nurses' station, Charge Nurse Denise Reed, her dark brown hair plaited into one long braid, smiles and hums as she cuts and bands together lengths of wide brown elastic used for strapping fetal monitors to the legs of laboring women.

Down the hall in Room 8, Nurse Jeanne Gates is rubbing the stomach of Melody Richards. The omnipresent Rebekah is, once again, telling Melody how selfless she is. Melody's sister Jamie, who is five months pregnant, Jamie's husband, Bobby, and their two-year-old daughter, Trisha Lea, and Student Nurse Deona Koth look on.

"I want candy," says Trisha Lea, suddenly. "I want candy! *Now!*"

In the midst of this mob lies the center of attention: Weeping Melody, swollen-breasted, huge-bellied, a wet washcloth on her forehead, sounds like the twelve-year-old she was often taken for, prepregnancy.

"Oh, they're hurting, they're hurting so *bad!*"

"They *told* you they would. Because they broke the membrane," snaps Rebekah. Recovering her sweetish tone of voice, she tells Melody once again how happy she's making others with her "act of love."

Nurse Jeanne Gates keeps rubbing Melody's stomach.

"Blow slowly," says the nurse. "Deep breaths!"

Melody blows slowly, takes deep breaths.

"Another deep breath," continues the nurse. "Good hard ones! Just the kind you need! It's on its way down!"

2210: 10:10 P.M.

In the recovery room, Zanna Morrison, still woozy from her anesthesia, lies smiling on the bed. She is watching her beloved nuzzle their tiny son. Sprawled catty-whompus in the chair, the new father is clad still in his disposable blue jumpsuit, curly blond hair peeking out now from under a baseball cap saying BOB'S ALL-TOYOTA WRECKING YARD. Shawn grins and sniffs his son's cheeks.

"He's so pretty! He looks just like his daddy!" says the young mother.

Nurse Jennifer Ostermeyer bustles around the room, taking Zanna's blood pressure, casting the occasional glance at the delighted new father.

"Can I ask you something?" says Zanna.

"Sure," says the nurse.

In a shy, small voice, Zanna worries aloud, asks a question surely asked (usually silently) by almost every new mother, rich or poor, sophisticated or simple, since there were mothers:

"I worry that the baby will stop breathing."

The nurse stops what she's doing, looks across to the young mother's face, and walks to the head of the bed, looking straight into Zanna's eyes.

"That's a very natural thing to worry about," she says without a hint of a smile. "I don't know what's going to happen to your baby in his life. But I can tell you that you have a healthy-looking baby. His color is fine, and he looks content."

"Do you really think so?" asks Zanna Morrison.

"Yes," answers the nurse. "I have a three-year-old myself. And sometimes, at night, I go into his room and put my hand on his sheet. Just to make sure he's breathing."

"Thank you," says the young mother, softly.

Quietly, the nurse, tall and smiling, leaves the new family alone.

CHAPTER SIX

The Nurse Wants a Baby

Nurses are often perceived as handmaidens to the doctor, as pale doctor wannabes. If they had the right stuff, they'd be doctors. (After all, why not go *all the way:* Why not be *a real doctor?*)

But ask Zanna Morrison, who will remember all her life how a tall nurse once cared for her on an April afternoon, how she gave comfort on the day Zanna's firstborn came into her life. It doesn't take much to see that doctors and nurses practice complementary, quite different, professions. Superficially, it might appear that the doctors get all the glory, while nurses get to do the dirty work: sponge-bathing sticky, cranky patients, bearing from hospital room reeking receptacles, pans chock-full of vomitus, urine, and feces. All the while wearing brave and beatific smiles. To be sure, it's the doctor who makes the slick and bloody incision, who stitches up the wound, who scribbles out the prescription for the antibiotics. But most of the direct care, most of the attention, most of the *healing* that happens in hospitals, comes from the nurse.

Zanna Morrison knows that, and she will remember Nurse

Jennifer Ostermeyer, and what she did for her, until the day she dies.

In our culture, as in the rest of Western civilization, women are directed to be the nurturers, the caregivers, expected to behave in traditional, gentle, "motherly" ways. To behave otherwise, to choose a profession long within the male purview—the law, say, or banking—is to assume "male" characteristics. Witness the "dress for success" code of the past decade or two, the injunction to jumped-up females to disguise their femaleness within male-cut suits, topped off with, if not a necktie, then at least one of those odd, stern silk neck bows.

The nurses working on 4NE are almost old-fashionedly feminine in appearance, pretty women with soft, long hair, their hip-swaying walks scarcely obscured by the baggy green or blue scrubs that are their uniforms. Their earlobes sport jewels, their fingernails are polished, their manner gentle.

Yet, among the nurses there's a toughness, a tensile strength, an ability to cope under the most desperate conditions. Daily and nightly, these graceful women soothe and comfort, counteract the frightening, emotionally dangerous sterility necessary in hospital rooms. It is the nurse who acts as buffer between doctor and patient.

Particularly in a teaching hospital, it is the nurse who is the patient's advocate, who stands beside the hapless bedridden soul, protecting the patient from the aggressor: an overeager medical student or resident determined to try out some just-learned skill, some new procedure or medication, some wondrous dazzlement of technology.

Then there are the patients, often angry, more often scared. There are always new things to learn, and residents who change every few months. (Nurturing those growing and learning M.D. egos is no picnic!) Long in their jobs, the nurses often find themselves (oh, so diplomatically) tutoring new doctors in the use of their newly acquired skills, and often, while they're at it, working in pointers on how not to lose it entirely during an emergency.

You can have a doctor freak out, and it's just like they're no use to you, thinks Jeanne Gates, R.N. Not that it hasn't happened to more than one nurse. There've been a couple of incidents up on Pill Hill's 4NE where the doctor's panicked. "Take her to the back! Take her to the back!" they'll say, insisting that the laboring woman needs an emergency c-section. And it's just like, well, *shit,* it takes ten minutes to get them to the back, and by the time you're there, they're fine. And you look at that paper strip and you go, "Why would you bring her back?" And the family's all upset, and it's like of no use to anybody. Jeanne isn't one to get ruffled easily, doesn't panic like a lot of people do. She doesn't call the doctor in for some kind of intervention until the baby's heart rate's been down for two or three minutes and she's tried everything. A lot of times, the doctor just gets in the way.

But it's nowhere near as bad here as at Fresno. There, it felt like doctors against the nurses, all the time. Jeanne saw her major role as a nurse there as a patient advocate, protecting the patient from the doctors.

Here, it's not like that at all. Not that there aren't a couple of the doctors more aggressive than others. But here, the residents help each other, they get along with each other, they get along with the nursing staff. There's just a whole lot of working together, and that's got to come from Dr. Kirk. He sets the tone for the way the doctors act, and what they're expected to do. As a matter of fact, the nursing staff has gotten a couple of very nice notes of appreciation from Dr. Kirk, praising them for the amount of work they do with the staffing they've got.

It's funny how life unfolds itself, one thing simply leading to another. Once upon a time, a young girl named Jeanne Elizabeth Aldrich thought she'd become a physical therapist, marry, have a batch of kids. Never, years ago, did Jeanne imagine she'd end up as a nurse, working with women giving birth, and hoping against hope that she'd finally get pregnant herself. Tomorrow she and Paul, her husband, have to go through a second artificial insemination procedure, separately. Paul will spend his time alone in a little room with a dog-eared *Playboy* or *Penthouse,* half the pictures already ripped out by the medical students peddling sperm to Pill Hill's sperm bank. (Young guys jerking their way through school, into anony-mous fatherhood, their manhood in one hand, stroke book in the other!)

Tomorrow before coming on her three-to-eleven shift, Jeanne—for her part in all this—will once again make weak jokes with Resident Jeff Jensen, who the first time didn't even recognize the nurse he'd been working with for months. Out of context, that's what she was. Jeanne had to remind him as he came at her with the syringe with the tiny squirt of Paul's essence. ("Hey, I *work* with you, remember?")

Jeanne Gates is twenty-eight and round, with sharp eyes and shiny dark hair and a soft, nervous laugh, a woman who doesn't miss anything going on around her. Born in Sacramento, she and her family moved to Hawaii when she was five. Her father worked for the phone company, and she went to a private school. At sixteen, and "into gymnastics" as was many an Olympics-watching young girl, one day her body went over the vault, but her knees stayed behind. The two years of physical therapy that followed piqued her interest in the PT profession. Her high school had a program where seniors could volunteer in a field that interested them, and that year Jeanne had liked her work in a couple of Honolulu hospitals. So she talked her father into letting her go to college on the mainland—as long as she could find a college that didn't cost much more than the University of Hawaii's in-state tuition.

California, where her grandparents still lived, had a good physical therapy program at Fresno State, and residency was simple enough to establish. She'd never even heard of Fresno before. All she could think of was cows. But it turned out to be a nice little city, even though it was very dry and sometimes very hot, getting up to 115 regularly. The school was real nice, beautifully landscaped, and after a period of really missing Hawaii, she came to really like the town. And she met Paul Henry Gates during her sophomore year. He was a true Californian—a winemaking major from Lodi, no less. In the end, she lived in Fresno for eight years.

With its status as a low-tuition state school, Fresno State is really popular, but their physical therapy program is very small, admitting only thirty-odd new students a year. Very, very picky they were, requiring a certain grade point average for admission, and an oral entrance interview as well as a written test. The year Jeanne applied, her more-than-respectable 3.55 GPA wasn't good enough. The lowest score

94

to be accepted into the PT program was 3.85, something like that. And she wasn't about to take those classes all over again to raise her grades. She didn't have it in her. Just forget it.

For a while Jeanne tried studying business—mostly because her father had always wanted her to—but she just couldn't see where it was going. Her direction had always been toward the health sciences. She tried hospital management. For a semester, she tried being a health sciences major. All along, her roommate was a nursing major who urged her to try nursing. But she'd never had a very glorified opinion of nurses. All those bedpans, and being bossed around by doctors and all. Her roomie kept at her, telling her that if she were a nurse she could fly in helicopters, or work in an emergency room, or in a doctor's office, or on an Indian reservation. So Jeanne thought, what the hell, she'd tried everything else.

The first semester of nursing school was really rough, with a lousy teacher. Jeanne hated it and was ready to drop out. She'd come home and cry. In her misery, she decided she'd give the second semester two weeks. But it was better, so she stuck with it.

In 1983, Jeanne—by then married two years to Paul Gates—graduated from California State University at Fresno. She'd already been working as a permittee for six months, having completed her course work and passed the state boards. Alas, there was a nationwide nursing glut, particularly severe in California, with radical cutbacks in welfare and MediCal, and resulting low censuses in hospitals. By the time Jeanne graduated, nothing in Fresno was open. Hating the thought of working in one, she even sank to applying at various nursing homes. Even they weren't hiring. So she ended up working in a tiny fifty-bed hospital in Dinuba, some twenty or thirty miles away from Fresno.

Dinuba is a Hispanic community populated by mostly agricultural workers. At Alta District Hospital, most of the doctors were GPs, general practitioners. Many people who came to the hospital, and the ones who worked there, had lived in the area all their lives. Alta was a general hospital that took care of just about everything, and Jeanne was hired as a medical surgical nurse. It was good practice, and she got her med-surg experience out of the way; six months later, she ended up at Valley Medical Center, the county hospital in Fresno.

She really liked the clientele, especially the Hispanic women, who are very sweet, very nice, very appreciative—completely different from a lot of the clients you get in L&D anywhere else. If they're from Mexico, they're very clean-living. They don't do drugs, they don't smoke, they don't drink. And they're just so appreciative of anything that you do for them.

Jeanne enjoys speaking Spanish and finds it is like a game to keep learning. Like the word "placenta," with that sharp enunciation Spanish has, the accent neatly placed on the center syllable: "*Pla-CEN-ta . . . pla-CEN-ta.*" The Hispanic men aren't so much fun to work with. At Fresno Jeanne saw a lot of them in the emergency room, after they'd been drinking or fighting or using drugs. They weren't as involved in their wives' labors as other ethnic groups are. Sometimes, they'd sit in the room with them. Sometimes they'd hold their hands. They're interested, you know, but they're not real pushy about it. They lag back, and you kind of have to involve them in what's going on. A lot of times, too, the husbands have to go back home and watch the other kids, and so they'd just leave their wives at the doorstep of the hospital and go. But for the wives, that's the way it is, the hardships of their life. They accept that.

It comes down to stereotypes, but a lot of it is true. Like Caucasians seem to be more demanding. Here on The Hill, you see lower income, a lot more welfare people. Jeanne tends to resent some of the Caucasian women more than she does the others, just because of all that demanding "you owe me" lah-de-dah stuff.

There are a lot of Hispanic girls that grew up here, or grew up in L.A. or whatever, they're the ones that are the prostitutes and doing drugs. Very seldom do you see a Hispanic woman who grew up in Mexico that does *anything*. The black population seems to fit pretty much into what the Caucasians do. They can be either nice and polite, or they can just be real demanding and rude, too.

Once in a while, Jeanne takes care of Hmong women, who retain much of their tribal customs from Southeast Asia. They have a lot of religious beliefs, or they did back in Fresno, when she was giving them a lot of care. They always wanted boys, for example, and they were completely disappointed, and it was the woman's fault, if it was a girl. And if it was a girl, they wanted the placenta, to tie a knot in the cord, because they didn't want any more of those! This was the end of the line, and they were going to tie a knot in that cord! The Hmong women never held their babies after they delivered them. They didn't even want to see them. Jeanne and the other nurses would fret about them bonding with their babies—and by the time you saw them the next day, they were taking care of their babies just fine. It's just that they don't want anything to do with them right after they're born—it's the father who holds them.

It was kind of hard to keep remembering what it was you were supposed to do, and not supposed to do. Like you don't touch the baby's head. And Hmongs don't look you in the eye. That's *rude*. If you're talking to them, it's rude to try to force eye contact. You never point at them. *That's* rude! We're so ingrained with whatever it is that we do in our own culture, we point at people, you look them in the eye all the time. Here on 4NE, you see some Hmong women, but not that often, and they usually have interpreters with them.

Jeanne doesn't reckon she's any more sensitive to ethnic minority patients than the other nurses on the floor. If you can speak any foreign language, she figures, you can identify with the patient more, understand what she's going through, simply because you know what she's saying.

While Jeanne's husband, Paul, finished up his winemaking degree and looked for a job, she continued working full time at Fresno's Valley Medical, and on top of that at a per-diem job at a private hospital. Paul applied all over—in Santa Rosa, the Napa area, in Stockton—but there were just too many winemakers per winery. Then he heard about a job at an Oregon winery, and applied for it. Jeanne was not happy about this. It was one of those bad times we all go through. She had just gone through painful surgery, part of an infertility workup, and her grandmother was dying. Then he came home and said he'd gotten the job, and they were moving. Go ahead, Jeanne told him, *I'm* not moving. For one thing, Paul had a pattern of keeping a job for three to six months, then quitting. And she had no interest, none at all, in living in Oregon.

Paul moved in July, having taken the job, and Jeanne finally joined him in October, once she was sure he wasn't going to quit that job as soon as she moved. In fact, he hung in there for almost a whole year, moving on to another winery job that paid twice as much. Now, he's with Veritas Winery, owned by OHSU's chief of radiology and his wife, a psychologist for the VA. After all these years, Paul now knows what it's like to work with doctors!

After the 1986 move, Jeanne was surprised to find she liked living in Oregon. Especially when they left Newberg, outside of Portland, to a house in the middle of the vineyard. It's nice, though being in the country and all, it gets kind of spooky at night, and it took some getting used to at first.

Almost from the start of their marriage, for some six and a half years now, Jeanne and Paul have been trying to have a baby. An earlier diagnosis in Fresno was less than revealing: Officially, the couple was experiencing "undiagnosed infertility." Swell. At first, naturally, Jeanne was the one who underwent extensive tests. Then, after the move to Oregon, she felt really fed up with all the uncomfortable, often painful, testing procedures. Let it rest a while, she figured, and just didn't think about it for a year or so. Finally, they went into OHSU's infertility services, and Paul was worked up. Really rough: She got the surgeries, he got to jerk off into a cup! Don't you *dare* complain to me, she would tell him.

Turned out Paul had an adequate sperm count, but the little buggers would just lie there and play dead—"poor motility," in fertility terms. So they put him on antibiotics for a couple of months. Finally, Jeanne and Paul were told they had a less than 10 percent chance of getting pregnant. And she was sick of the surgeries.

What they finally decided to do, even though there was only a small chance of it working, was to try artificial insemination, but using Paul's sperm. So it's back to mutilated *Penthouses* for Paul, and for Jeanne, lying on her back while some resident injects the result into her cervix, using a catheter off an IV set. Lie still for fifteen minutes, and wish you were comfortable enough with the situation to say some smartassy thing to the resident. Like, "Shall I light up a cigarette?" Or maybe, "Was it good for you?"

Funny. Yearning as much as she does for her own baby, it doesn't really bother Jeanne to work with the pregnant women on L&D. What gets to her is when the people she *knows* get pregnant. It's a little depressing, though you'd think she'd get used to it. In the six years she and Paul have been trying for a baby, it seems like everyone they know has been pregnant twice. Paul likes to crack jokes, likes to tell Jeanne it's all her fault. That she has bad eggs.

With all the jokes, there's always an underlying tension. She's told him she won't go through the surgery again, and he just won't talk about the other options, the test-tube stuff and GIFT—the gamete interfallopian transfer. With the in vitro, test-tube baby, procedure, they have to do a laparoscopy to harvest the eggs, and then perform another one to implant them back, fertilized, into you. It costs $5,000, and they certainly can't come up with that. No insurance company is going to cover it. Anyway, with only a 20 percent chance of it even working, it's just like ridiculous. Jeanne can't believe people actually pay for it.

The other thing is adoption. Paul's totally against adopting, and that really bothers her. He says you don't know what the kid's parents were like, you know, like what drugs they did, what their lifestyle was like, and stuff like that. He says he doesn't want some idiot's kid, but Jeanne wants a baby, period. Adopting one, though, costs something like $10,000, or else you wait forever and ever. So that's why they're doing this with the tattered *Penthouse*s.

One of Paul's last visits to the doctor, it really hit him hard. He went by himself. The doctor came in and had the wrong chart, kept insisting that Paul had lost a lot of weight. Paul says, "No..." And the doctor says, "Yeah, you've lost quite a *bit* of weight!" And Paul says, "No—actually, I've put *on* a few pounds!" And finally the dumb doctor realizes he's got the wrong patient and the wrong chart, and he comes back in with the right chart and says, "Well, basically you just can't have *kids*!" Just like that, real rude. And when Jeanne gets home from work that night, Paul is dead drunk. Drunk and very preoccupied. He needs to talk about it, and *now*, he says. It's okay with him to try the donor sperm, Paul says.

Jeanne's talked with him about that. She was surprised to

find it doesn't bother him at all. In fact, it bothers her more. The reason Jeanne feels funny about AID—artificial insemination by donor—is that she can say very mean things sometimes when she gets mad. She can be very bitchy. And she's afraid that later, if they had a kid from AID, she might say something in the middle of a fight like, "So it isn't your kid, *anyway!*" She hopes she wouldn't, but you just never know. Sometimes Jeanne says things that are *intended* to be mean, and they certainly come across that way.

Paul is a lot different from her, almost the opposite, nice and easygoing most of the time. He puts up with a lot—stresses from work and so on. He has his quirks, too, so they kind of even out. He does seem to do okay with this baby thing, unless he's been drinking, and then he gets a little upset. Like, what do you tell people? Do you tell people? Do you just keep it to yourselves? What do you say to parents—his parents—if anything? Paul doesn't get along so well with his parents, anyway, so he doesn't want to tell them anything, nothing at all.

CHAPTER SEVEN

DAY 3: Wednesday, April 13

("She's so goddamned fucking beautiful!" says the father, resplendent in baseball cap.)

1500: 3:00 P.M.

BY AMTRAK THE JOURNEY from Salt Lake City, Utah, to Portland, Oregon, takes just minutes shy of seventeen hours, and at three o'clock this afternoon, Mary Fran Bidwell and her husband, Jack, are just two hours from Portland's Union Station. Having boarded the train at ten minutes to midnight, they sat up all night, holding hands. They had told themselves they would try to sleep, but they are excited beyond sleep. Tomorrow, April 14, will be the day they meet their new son. After they left Salt Lake, knowing the baby was about to be born, they called the hospital each time the train stopped.

When they called during a stop in Ogden, at 12:43, they learned that Melody Richards (whose name the Bidwells don't know) was still in labor. But when they called from Pocatello, Idaho, at 3:10, they learned they were the new parents of a healthy baby son, born an hour and a half earlier, at 1:40.

Daniel Thomas George Bidwell will be his name. The "Thomas" and "George" after their own fathers, the "Daniel" because it's the kind of all-purpose name that will last him a lifetime. He can be "Danny" as a little boy—clear through high school, even—"Dan" as a grown man, and if Heavenly Father sees fit, one day he may even be "Old Daniel."

Only a couple more hours till the train pulls into Union Station, where Mary Fran's cousin Sue will pick them up and take them to her house. The hospital wants them to wait until tomorrow to see him. Then, finally—finally!—they'll hold their baby in their arms!

Mary Fran and Jack have been married seven years next month, and they have never used any form of birth control, not even once. They were virgins when they met at Brigham Young University, and went steady all through college, vowing not to make love all the way until they were married. They almost made it, too—then, three weeks before their wedding, in the backseat of Jack's car, they just got completely carried away.

The newlyweds fretted all the way through their honeymoon, worried that their blunder might have gotten their family started embarrassingly early. Then, the night before they were to leave the borrowed condo on Waikiki, they found out that Mary Fran wasn't pregnant, after all. They were, of course, relieved. Now, seven years later, they realize it would have been more than okay if she had gotten pregnant that night, or any other of the probably hundreds of times they've made love on their marriage bed.

Jack Bidwell works for his father, managing the lumberyard begun at the turn of the century by his grandfather. Mary Fran teaches second grade, but now that they have a baby, she's going to stop work. A baby needs a full-time mother. And Danny is going to get the best mother she can be.

Oh, Danny!

1547: 3:47 P.M.

It is a good thing Jack and Mary Fran Bidwell are not in the INCU nursery in Pill Hill's L&D right now. Melody Richards's sister Jamie, herself five months pregnant with her second child, is holding her sister's newborn son. Crooning to

102

him, she is kissing him, sniffing his cheeks. Most of all, Jamie is trying not to cry.

Jamie Ferguson is, when you get right down to it, actively engaged in what is currently referred to as "bonding" with her robust nephew. Her feelings for this little boy are ferocious, almost violent. She keeps having to resist the urge to chomp a big bite out of one of his fat pink cheeks.

Early on in her pregnancy, Melody had asked Jamie if she and Fred would consider adopting the baby. Their reaction had been one of undisguised horror. After all, Trisha Lea wasn't more than a year and a couple of months old at the time. And then, when Melody asked a second time, Jamie was already a month or so along with this one. So no seemed like the right answer, the only answer. But now, she isn't sure. In fact, the only thing Jamie Ferguson is sure of is that she loves this baby, almost as much as if he were her own.

That scene when the baby was finally born! Boy, was Melody in labor a long, long time! And finally, hours after Fred took Trisha Lea home, it was just Melody, looking like she was twelve, crying and pushing for all she was worth, and that obnoxious bitch—what's her name?—oh yeah, Rebekah from the Ward—who kept saying how "selfless" Melody was to be giving up her baby, and that she wasn't to even *look* at it when it got born.

And then, he was born. The girl doctor with the freckles, Dr. Delaplain, pregnant with her own belly sticking out to here, was the one who delivered Melody's kid. She did that part where they cut you to make room for the baby's head coming out. And then Melody gives one huge push, like she was making doody, and *out he comes,* kind of oozing right into the doctor's hands. That Rebekah (who will not shut up about how she's got seven kids) gets all woozy-looking, kind of falling backward a little, then she pushes the nurse out of the way and tells that girl doctor for about the ten millionth time she's not supposed to show the baby to Melody.

Melody by this time is bawling her head off, just saying over and over, "Is it a *girl*? Is it a *boy*?"

And that doctor, she says something like, "Here's your son, Melody!" and puts him right onto her chest, just like that.

And Melody gets all sappy then and keeps kissing him and patting him all over his sticky little body. And she doesn't even flinch when they have to push down hard on her stomach. Boy, that Rebekah looks fit to kill, like she's going to slap that pregnant doctor, who is sort of humming and smiling as she sews Melody back up down there.

Melody's sister Jamie rocks the baby while she feeds him his bottle. ("Matthew," she thinks. "Matthew is a good name!")

Observing all this, the INCU nurses exchange looks.

In the rocking chair, a few feet from Jamie and her nephew, two-day-old crack addict Timothy Edwards squeaks atonally as the beautiful freckly-faced nurse named Mary tries (again, to no avail) to get him to suck from the bottle.

As her sister is merrily bonding away with the small boy in 4NW, Melody Richards is weeping softly over in South Hospital, about as far away from the new mothers and babies as you can get without falling off Marquam Hill into the Willamette River.

"Yeah, I think I made the right decision," she keeps telling the nurses and anybody else who'll listen to her. "I just didn't think it was going to feel this way...."

Then she starts talking about how she's only eighteen, after all, and about how she has her whole life ahead of her, and about how she can always have more kids. And about how these people who are coming by train from Utah had to borrow a whole lot of money for a new house so they could have a special room for the baby, and a yard.

1612: 4:12 P.M.

Fili, the hospital aide, has emptied the trash cans outside the two operating rooms on 4NE, and is mopping the hallway floor.

On the wall behind the nurses' station, The Board shows every single L&D room filled.

Wanda Servoss—twenty, unmarried, and accompanied by her best-girlfriend-since-grade-school—is in the PAR, normally used just for recovery, waiting for a regular labor and delivery room.

Luanne Schmidt, twenty-five and black, is in Room 18, holding hands with her husband, who is looking forward to the arrival of their third child.

In Room 16, a thirteen-year-old named Dawna Hawkins tells her sister that she doesn't care what they have to do to her, as long as they get that *thing* out of her.

In Room 10, Linda Brown has been brought upstairs to be prepared for a c-section. Linda has been tucked into a bed in the Mother-Baby Unit for five weeks now, thanks to a *chronic abruption:* Her baby's placenta is tearing away from the wall of the uterus, and Linda has been bleeding mildly. With this abruption, the chances for intrauterine growth retardation are significant. After an amniocentesis showed the baby's lungs to be mature, the doctors conferred. The baby being thirty-three weeks, probably weighing in at almost four pounds, they reckon it's all right for her to come out and join her parents.

In Room 8, a sallow, thin nineteen-year-old named Faye Leaper, in her forty-third week of pregnancy, is wishing it were all over. Or, even better, that it had never happened. Glumly, she uses the remote control to zap the TV, finally settling for cartoons.

In Room 2, Jolene Winegard, a plump twenty-five-year-old private patient of Dr. Amanda Clark, rests up from the breech birth of her second child, a daughter. Her red-haired, freckled husband, a tall, heavyset man in his forties, slumps back in his armchair, looking far more drained than his wife.

In the Exam Room, there's Nurse-Midwife patient Patti Rausch, who (counting her knee-high argyles of tan, red, and green) probably outweighs her adjacent, anxious husband by fifty pounds. She shares the tiny room with a falsely laboring woman in her forties who will soon be sent back home.

Jeffrey Rausch can't get over the fact that Patti insisted on wearing those argyle socks tonight. She's sure she was wearing them the night she knows they did it for this kid. ("They'll bring us luck!" she kept hollering from the living room sofa after her water broke this morning. "Jeffie, I am *not* going to that frigging hospital until you find those frigging socks!" He finally found them—one in the dryer, the other all balled up and covered with cat hair, under the bed. *Women!*)

A tiny black woman, thirty-two weeks pregnant and perhaps in her mid-twenties, long hair ornately plaited into corn-rows, sits in a wheelchair in the hall beside the nurses' station. Rocking her body back and forth, back and forth, she presses a wet paper towel to her bleeding nose. She's in, she says, because her boyfriend beat her up. Her *ex*-boyfriend.

In Special Delivery, Marianne Buskirk, a twenty-three-year-old with poreless ivory skin, her pale blond hair frantically frizzed by what she calls "the $9 Permanent from Hell," is pushing as hard as she can. A private patient of The Hill's nurse-midwifery practice, she's being coached by Nurse-Midwife Carol Howe.

"*Breathe,* honey," says Marianne's husband, Ray, a short, balding man with a wispy little blond moustache. His baseball cap reads SNAP-ON TOOLS, and he's clad in Levi 501s and a faded red plaid flannel shirt with rolled-up sleeves revealing a tattoo permanently proclaiming what turned out, after all, to be a fleeting and beer-sodden alliance to a woman named SHERILYN.

"*Breathe!*" he repeats with enthusiasm.

One more good push. Out comes a hulking 9¾ pound girl named Tiffany Michelle who looks like she should be wearing boxing gloves. Apgar: 9.

"Oh, God!" says Tiffany Michelle's daddy, starting to sob. "Oh, God!" He kisses his wife on her damp, flushed cheek. The two of them start to laugh.

"She's just so goddamned fucking *beautiful!*" says Ray Buskirk.

"Honey!" singsongs his wife from her bed. "Don't talk like that in front of the K-I-D!"

They all laugh: the mother, the father, the two nurse-midwives, the tall, angular nurse, and the nurse-midwifery student.

Tiffany Michelle blinks and looks around, then begins to scream very, very loud.

"Oh boy," says her father. "Oh boy, oh boy, oh boy!"

*   *   *

Hilary Blanchard, barricaded in her room on the third-floor Mother-Baby Unit, scowls as she leafs through a copy of *Architectural Digest,* pausing to take an occasional sip from the stubby bottle of Perrier on the table beside her. God. The smell of the meat loaf, potatoes, and green beans that were carried into the other patient rooms at lunchtime made her want to puke, even with the door slammed shut.

Two hours and seventeen minutes have passed since Hilary got today's massage. Tanned, with elegant facial lines, Hilary's mother sits alongside her supine daughter with the tentative pregnancy. She knits silently on a pullover in an elaborate fisherman's knit design. The *click-click-click* of maternal needles provides a quiet counterpoint to the occasional *swish* of magazine pages turning. Richie was supposed to run by Briggs & Crampton to pick up dinner for both Hilary and her mother tonight. He was supposed to come by first.

Hilary wishes he'd hurry up. She's been working on the unicorn for hours, and had forgotten how it took her mother eons to do one lousy pillowtop. Sighing ostentatiously, she picks up today's *New York Times* and has another bash at the crossword. Thirty-eight across: *Suffix with velvet.* With the fine nib of her gold Cross pen, Hilary prints in EEN. Thirty-nine across: *Associate.* Easy! PARTNER. Forty-one across: *Legume.* Seven letters. Starts with s...can't be PEANUT. What is it? Shit! Hilary throws the folded newspaper across the room, just as a nurse comes through the door.

Unseen by her daughter, the older woman exchanges glances with the impassive-faced nurse. With subtle shrug of cashmere-sweatered shoulders, Hilary's mother rolls her eyes.

The nurse smiles.

On the surface, in these circumstances, Hilary Blanchard may look like a spoiled brat, a resentful kid forced to pay a higher price for her toys than the other kids. Without question, this young woman is a Yuppie, a well-educated, well-bred, upper-middle-class American whose life needs a biological child to be complete. Again without question, Hilary has never served five minutes of what has come to be called "street time."

Much has been made of America's "baby lust" in recent years. Wanting to have it all—wanting career, marriage, house, two cars—today's men and women have postponed child-bearing until all the accoutrements of the well-appointed life have been firmly set into place. As it has turned out, and for a variety of complex reasons, "having it all" has turned out to be more difficult than the shiny promises. One in six American couples is officially diagnosed as "infertile," a statistic that includes those with earlier, elective tubal ligations and vasectomies whose changed lives and different partners have caused them to switch their votes on parenthood.

At the moment you are reading this, ten million Americans are struggling, without immediate success, to have children. Begetting a child has become a complex and controversial project, the technologies for "alternative" conception leaping forward with space-age speed while the ethical, moral, religious, and legal issues shuffle along behind, as though on foot.

For both men and women, it is more than understandable, this desire to have a child of one's own. When William Stern and his wife, Elizabeth, made the decision that led to the birth of Baby M, his motivation, it was said, was in part prompted by his stated need to "continue his bloodline." Stern, at least, was fertile. Yet men who are infertile do not have the option of hiring a "surrogate's" womb for nine months. Their choice is childlessness or adoption.

Like the barren woman, the infertile man is likely to regard his body as damaged, inadequate, incapable of carrying on the species. His self-esteem, self-image, and sense of inadequacy are stirred into the emotional mix. While women are perhaps more focused on pregnancy and giving birth, for the infertile man the irrevocable loss may be that ineffable sense—that reality—of a family line continued, one generation unfolding into the next, and the next, and the next.

Dare we call it immortality? Some richly textured sense of personal continuity, comes—Ah! Perhaps *only* comes!—with the having of children, with your children having children, and their children continuing your line. Surely, there is something gut-wrenching, wonderful, glorious in knowing that, a century and more down the road, a nimble-fingered someone you'll never meet may cast yarn onto a knitting needle in exactly the fashion your grandmother taught you, in the way you, in your time on this planet, instructed your own small, clumsy-fingered daughters. Sometime in the mists of the future, will the secret way to dovetail a cherrywood box be revealed by yet another careful father, to yet another eager, freckle-faced son?

Who knows such things? Something sweetly soothes in knowing that an odd cast of feature—a nose? a pair of deep-set hazel eyes? a loping walk?—will be carried on. As each generation marches forth, it totes along the rackety, clumsy burden of family eccentricities. With luck, with any luck at all, even values you cherish in the late twentieth century may wend their way intact, purely and cleanly into the next century.

Man or woman, what could be more natural than wanting a child of one's own? Denied this in the natural course of events, that wanting can move swiftly to a yearning, and thence to despair. The yearning desperation for a baby has been likened to hunger, to feeling lost, to a sense of being uninvited to the human party. Baby-craving, as most of us have seen—or experienced—can cause a life to go askew, can create a rift in the once-happy marriage. Can give birth itself to feelings of resentment between husband and wife, between the fertile and infertile halves of a couple.

It is a primal need, this wanting of a child. One that often boils down to a dangerous, heartbreakingly simple edict: *Give me a child, or I will find someone who can!*

Once progeny has been, in whatever manner, acquired, styles of parenthood would appear to pattern themselves after styles of living. A sort of sociological ontology recapitulating phylogeny. And many of today's would-be American parents don't merely want a child. They want Designer Kids, children assembled to their own specifications. In search of a child of the "right" gender, fertile parents trek to clinics to be artificially inseminated with their own viable sperm, which has been treated to help predetermine the gender of their coming attraction.

It sometimes seems that late-twentieth-century America has succeeded in a sort of Yuppification of parenthood. Put bluntly, children viewed in passing often appear to be ornaments, possessions evidently acquired to accessorize the well-appointed life. A life that includes the house and cars, the appropriate apparel, the hot tub, the VCRs—and, of course, the two careers.

There is something chilling in the spectacle of two-year-old boys toddling along in blue Oxford-cloth dress shirts like Daddy's, identical right down to the button-down collar. While in expensive toy stores "thirtysomething" parents hotly debate which stuffed animal will harmonize best with the carefully arranged ambiance of the living room, glittering beads of drool festoon cunning little Izod polo shirts. Children who can't even walk yet dangle tiny feet shod in Nike "running" shoes from their sleekly designed Italian strollers.

But the "I-want-it-all-and-I-want-it-*now*" mentality of the youngish and upwardly mobile dovetails neatly with that genuinely heartfelt urge to procreate. An urge that, in Hilary Blanchard's case, is finally being satisfied in a public hospital atop a hill in Portland, Oregon.

And so she lies in a hospital bed, this young and unhappy woman in her awkward *accouchement,* shuddering at the sounds she hears beyond her door, leafing through her magazines, poking her tapestry needle through the canvas depicting the captive unicorn, waiting. Waiting for the elegant, flower-strewn meals to be delivered. Waiting for the masseuse to arrive. Waiting for the friends to call and shake their heads at the horrible room in the horrible hospital.

Hilary Blanchard knows the wait will be worth it, because she will, in the end, have the child.

CHAPTER EIGHT

(Some want babies, some don't.)

ON PILL HILL, THE patients aren't the only women yearning for children. Third-Year Resident Julie Bouchard, thirty, looking over The Board on the wall of the nurses' station, makes no bones about the fact that she's been trying since November to get pregnant. That's when she went off the pill. Sometimes it gets pretty comical.

Last night, Julie knew she was ovulating, but she was on call, so she and Glenn planned a little tryst right upstairs in one of the residents' sleeping rooms. They just took the mattress and put it on the floor and went at it. And everybody, everybody, everybody knew about it.

Some people are just more fun to tease than others—and is Julie ever getting it since last night! With her bright, sparkly eyes and long dark shag haircut and thin, nervous energy, the would-be-pregnant resident is fair game for good-natured ribbing from the nurses and other residents.

Like all the other residents, Julie came to Pill Hill to do her OB/GYN residency through a sort of an intense, computer-arranged marriage, one that will last for four years. With The Match, as it's called, you go around and interview at different teaching hospitals around the country. You send out applications, do your interviews, then put together a list of places you want to go, rating them on a scale of 1 through 10. Each residency program rates the applicants who applied and were interviewed, and it all goes into a computer. And then one day—in Julie's case, the thirteenth of March, 1985—future doctors all around the country find out where they'll be serving out their residencies. If you haven't matched up, you find out the day before, and enter the phone competition for places that haven't matched up with new residents.

Julie was the first highly educated person in her family. Her mother worked in an office, her father was employed by a textile company, managing quality control. Her sister went on to college, and that was a big deal, too. The way Julie tells it, she herself was "kind of a bum," into having fun, period, after her 1975 graduation from high school in Piscataway, a central New Jersey commuter town handy to New York City. In her graduating class of six hundred, she graduated number five, despite seventy days of absence during her senior year.

After two years of post–high-school fooling around, Julie Bouchard decided to go to one of those medical-assistant schools, the ones you hear about on the radio. (GET A CAREER IN SIX MONTHS! CALL THIS NUMBER NOW!) She got a job in a private pediatrician's office. For a year and a half, Julie steered young patients and their mothers into the examination rooms, gave injections, ran simple lab tests, doing simple nursing duties in addition to scheduling appointments and answering the phones. She was struck by what she saw, admiring the doctors, envying them their daily challenges.

One day, it just hit her: That's what *I'm* going to do! So she applied to Rutgers University in New Brunswick, right there next to Piscataway, beginning eight long years through undergraduate school and medical school. Obstetrics and gynecology appealed to her almost immediately. The specialty was her favorite rotation in med school, and she really liked the people she met. These were the kind of people she wanted to be, with a better attitude toward patients than other doctors seemed to have.

Surgeons, she observed, seemed colder, wanting only to operate, caring less about the patient per se. The internal-medicine types? Well, all they seemed to do was think about their patients in a sort of mental masturbation way. (The joke goes like this: Why are internists like fleas? Because they're the last thing to leave a dying dog.) And with OB/GYN, you have a lot of healthy patients, women who tend to be a little more compliant. A nonpregnant patient may have high blood pressure but feels okay and doesn't want to take her medication. But when you're pregnant, you have a big reason to take what's been prescribed for you.

But residency! You just have no idea what it's like until you're in it. Even though she went through med school and worked with tons of residents, she never quite understood the intensity, the lack of sleep, the responsibility of it all. *And that mind-numbing fatigue.*

University hospitals tend to be the old county hospitals, like this one. Some places, like L.A., still have old county hospitals, and deal with just an indigent population. In Portland there are a lot of white people, and so few minorities. Though The Hill handles more minorities than anyplace else in the city, they hardly see any. At least in comparison with what Julie Bouchard was used to on the East Coast. Lots more black and Puerto Rican people.

When she's done, Julie thinks she'd like to go into private practice. Not that she'd mind a university setting. Portland's probably out, though. Friends who finished their residency last year went out and opened a practice here, and they're hardly making it. You can always deliver babies, of course, but they're just not doing any gynecology. Instead of paying off old debts and making money, they're getting in deeper, borrowing money to pay for new equipment for their office! You can go to towns not far from Portland and do a lot better. Even places like Oregon City, fifteen, twenty miles away.

Seven years ago, Julie finally married Glenn Beyerman, her sweetheart all the way back to high school days in Piscataway. He's an environmental engineer, specializing in hazardous waste, and that's what he'd *like* to be doing right now. But while Julie finishes up her residency, Glenn has been working in the city's industrial waste water department, issuing permits, making sure people comply with regulations about what goes into sewers.

Glenn's been wonderful wonderful wonderful. Very supportive, as the saying goes. The marriage could never have survived if he wasn't independent, willing to fill time by himself. He knows better than to sit around and wait for Julie to get home. Either she doesn't come home, or she comes home tired and in a bad mood. He knows how to keep himself busy. They just appreciate the time they have together. When they were in college, they kind of staggered who went to school. Like he went to the New Jersey Institute of Technology for two years while Julie was off two years, then he took a year and a half off while she went. Only one semester did they go to school at the same time.

Julie's parents are real proud of her. They have this vague notion that she works a lot. But they really don't have any concept of how much she does, what her responsibilities are. And you just can't explain that.

Like last week. There was a baby that died. And then a girl, a young woman who'd just had a baby, died. A sixteen-year-old girl Julie had been taking care of. That was terrible. And Dr. Kirk has always made a big thing about how you handle fetal and maternal demise, about what you do when babies and mothers die on you, no matter how hard you try. There isn't any specific training as such about it, but everyone has been sensitized to these deaths. Nick—Nicholas Abrudescu, who everyone thinks is so cool and distant—he was the one who put his arms around Julie while she cried about the girl dying. This girl, this sixteen-year-old, went home after having her baby and had sex right away, and air got into her vagina and worked its way up, and she got an embolus, an air bubble in her bloodstream, and it killed her. Just the saddest thing.

Dr. Kirk was in a meeting and couldn't respond to the code calling him to 4NE. But that afternoon, he hand-wrote a note to the despondent resident:

Julie—
    It is never easy when you lose a patient and maternal deaths in many ways are the most difficult.
    We would not be "real" doctors if these events did not affect us but take heart in knowing that your

patients have been receiving fine care, you are doing an excellent job and your natural talents for our specialty are evident.

Thank you,
Paul

Julie was really happy that Dr. Kirk wrote her. You don't get a whole lot of positive reinforcement around here, but you do get negative reinforcement. People let you know when you do something they don't like.

The nurses, though, are great here. The best. They know how to deal with doctors and residents really well. Say a brand-new intern comes in, fresh out of med school, and doesn't know anything. Well, the nurse who's been working here several years knows how to read a strip, knows what to do in a particular situation. She may not know all the pharmacologic and physiologic basis for everything like a doctor does, but *she knows*.

The nurse knows what needs to be done, she helps you out a lot. And the nurses really know how to do that without belittling the interns. They're just also the best at picking up problems, at identifying and fixing them.

It's been over five months since Julie and Glenn have been trying to get pregnant. It was like they expected it to happen just like *that*! when she went off the pill. When it didn't, it was so depressing. Now they're at the point where they have to time things just right, figure out when she's ovulating. Like that business last night, when she and Glenn had to, ahem, take advantage of Julie's ovulating while on call. Not exactly moonlight and roses, but what the hell. Everybody's still razzing her about it. There aren't a lot of secrets when you're in residency together.

Everybody around here thinks those movies and TV shows about doctors and residents sleeping around are pretty ridiculous. You don't even have time to sleep with your own spouse! What the residents want is sleep, period. And if Julie and Glenn have a baby nine months from now, in January of the new year, everyone will know when the date of conception was, that's for sure! If it works—when it works—Julie will take off six weeks, then have the baby in child care for a few months.

And next year, she'll be a chief resident and that's lots easier than the first three years. And between residency and a job, Glenn and Julie and the baby can travel, maybe go to Europe.

Even while trying so hard to get pregnant, it doesn't bother her to see all the babies born around here. What really gets her are the abortions you do in the clinic downstairs, or downtown in other clinics. Some of the residents moonlight in those clinics, doing abortions, and a couple of times Julie's gone because they needed people. That's a little bit bothersome. More than a little bit, in fact. Before she was trying for a baby, it bothered her, but not in the same way. The ones that are hard are the ones that are further along than just D&Cs. They look like babies. Or pieces of babies.

You see a fair number of dead babies, ones that are born too early to make it or whatever. It's something you get used to, but it's never good. The first couple of times, it's very hard just knowing what to say to the parents. Another hard part is there's so much incest, so much sexual abuse resulting in pregnancy for these very young girls.

Julie has a patient who's nineteen or twenty, and she's been pregnant eight times. She has only one child from all these pregnancies, a kid who's a year and a half old. The rest were self-induced abortions. She told Julie she beat herself on the stomach until she'd lose the baby! And you ask her about sexual abuse, and she says, *Oh yeah, my father abused me, some of those pregnancies were from him.*

Meanwhile, the guy that had come in with her this time was in his fifties, really sleazy-looking. Turns out he's not her father, he's the father of the baby she's carrying now. And who has custody of that one-and-half-year-old? Her father, who made her pregnant, is now taking care of her child. His daughter and his granddaughter, the same baby. Telling all this to Julie, her doctor, doesn't faze this young woman, not one little bit.

Third-Year Resident Julie Bouchard realizes she's been staring at The Board for a couple of minutes now. All these women, here to have babies some of them don't even want in the first place. Who are they? Where do they come from? In Room 2, Jolene Winegard, Mandy Clark's private patient...

116

Patti Rausch, in the Exam Room . . . Dawna Hawkins, the thirteen-year-old in Room 16.

Nobody's really heating up too much yet. A cup of coffee sounds good. Maybe there are some cookies in the coffee/ supply room. For some reason, Julie's feeling a little stomach-achy today.

1715: 5:15 P.M.

Dawna Hawkins and her older sister, LaTreesha, are watching television in Room 16. Pa Ingalls is giving Laura some kind of stern lecture about helping her mother with something.

LaTreesha came in with Dawna on Thursday night. The hospital people acted real surprised that thirteen-year-old Dawna was in labor, on account of her only being six months along. But they poked her all kinds of places (Dawna *hates* that part), and they said, Sure enough, this baby's on the way. But then they went and stuck her in a room in another part of the hospital and tried to keep the baby from coming. What difference did it make *when* the baby comes, anyway? Long as you got to have it anyhow, why not get it over with?

But it was boring in that dumb room downstairs, and even though all of them tried to keep the baby from getting itself born, it started up again. Her sister was just then finishing painting Dawna's toenails this great color, a kind of a light pinky-purple that looked real good with her dark skin. And she was fixing to take all that chewed-up red polish off of her fingernails and give them a coat of the purple when *pow!*, Dawna gets this really bad pain, and her sister runs out to get the nurse. So they put her on this kind of bed with wheels on it and shove it into an elevator and down the halls, right as she's about to get some lunch, not that the food is so hot, and here she been all day with not a bite to eat, nothing. (Breakfast was real pukey-looking, and she wasn't about to eat *that* shit!)

Dawna's bag of waters is full and tight, and she has to take a shit, and they won't let her. They're trying to tell her that if she sits and goes, that'll do something to the curd or quarter or something, they tell her, so they're going to cut a

117

little hole inside to let some of the water out, and that'll make the baby come down more. They say it isn't going to hurt none, but she doesn't believe them.

"I don't care," Dawna says, when they explain what they need to do. "Just get that thing out of me."

Out by the nurses' station, someone congratulates Charge Nurse Denise Reed on her pregnancy. A shadow briefly crosses her lovely, open face. She tugs at her long, glossy braid.

"Oh, I guess you didn't hear. I had a miscarriage," says the nurse, smiling tightly.

"Ah, Denise—I'm so sorry! If I'd known . . . " The voice trails off.

"That's okay," says Denise. "It'll work eventually. How're your kids doing?"

Denise Reed hopes it will all work out eventually. Timing is everything. In a way, it's probably a good thing she's not having a baby just now. After all, Andy's still in school, and she'd be like a single parent. Once he gets into medical school, even though things will be just as hard, there won't be that pressure to make it.

When you think about it, it's a wonder Denise got pregnant in the first place. With Andy full time at Portland State, then working night shift in the ER here, their schedules aren't coordinated. Sometimes it seems like they exist in parallel worlds, yearning, viewing each other through a huge pane of glass. Since Denise works the three-to-eleven-P.M. shift, he'll come up to 4NE on his way to work, and if it isn't too busy, they go into the stairwell and chat. (And neck, if nobody's coming up the stairs or going down!) Otherwise, they just have something like ten minutes together on Wednesday evenings, and every other weekend.

Denise is thirty-one. She met Andy Reed when he was a paramedic student, rotating through L&D. Their eyes met, and it was lust at first sight! He's so nice, and so cute, and they married last June.

Aside from not being able to spend much time with her husband, Denise likes this shift fine. And she likes the work, especially the fast pace and doing the operating room stuff. You never know what's going to happen when you come to work. Sometimes you can just be sitting at a bedside, doing lots of support for a laboring woman. Other times you do the high-tech stuff. Then other times you're just flying up and down that hall, making sure that everything's being taken care of. Her favorite part is seeing the babies come out. That she can be there every time, it's just such a wonderful, wonderful gift.

Denise Benhard grew up in California, with her special-education-teacher mother and her little sister, in the foothills of the Sierras in Grass Valley. As a student at Mills College, she studied pre-med, partly because the school had a very good rate of getting their pre-meds into medical school. As she was ending her years at Mills, she saw what horrible pressure it could be—a couple of her classmates who married in their senior year ended up getting divorced soon after, in med school, and there was even one suicide. So she took another look and decided to put off taking the MCAT, the Medical College Admission Test.

In 1979, the day after she graduated from Mills, Denise came up to Oregon on a lark, and decided to stay. Soon she was working on a master's degree in biology, but got interested in nursing instead. Working as a nurse's aide at Portland's Providence Hospital, helping with profoundly brain-damaged kids, she was shocked at the way nurse's aides are treated, the kind of hierarchy and roles that exist. But oh, how she loved the kids!

After Mills College, nursing school at OHSU was a shock. She thought many of the classes were horrible. But she stuck it out, graduating in 1983.

For the next two years, Denise worked in OHSU's Surgical Intensive Care Unit. She liked it, but it was hard. Patients died all the time. Here on L&D, people usually do pretty well. They have labor, they get a baby, and their only problems are real up-front kinds of "social problems." But there are trade-offs. In SICU it was wonderful. There was every piece of equipment you could want, everything was so organized, great staffing. It was run tremendously. On 4NE it's always scattered, always short-staffed, with patients in the halls. It's not Dr. Kirk's fault. It's just that L&D is stuck over here in North Hospital, with no ancillary services set up nearby to support it. It makes it hard to take care of the very ill patients. The intensive care units—for both mothers and their babies—are way over in South Hospital, which is too far away.

Evening Charge Nurse Denise Reed tries to keep a handle on what everyone's condition is, so that patient loads are well distributed for safe patient care. She tries to maintain a good working environment for the nurses, tries to work with the physicians so that big mistakes aren't made, like accepting five transports from other hospitals at once. And she works with patients herself. What she really likes is working with the intensively ill patients.

All things considered, Denise Reed thinks it's okay not to have a baby right now. Her time will come.

2015: 8:15 P.M.

Nurse Carolyn Bachhuber tells Dawna Hawkins that an old wives' tale says that if the heartbeat is on the high side, it'll be a girl. Her baby's heart is beating pretty fast, she says, so that must mean she will have a daughter soon.

"I could care less," is Dawna's muttered reply.

"What?" asks the nurse.

"Nuthin'," says the patient. "I didn't say *nuthin'*!"

Dawna and her sister are watching television. On the screen suspended on the window wall of Room 16 is *The Bell Jar,* a movie based on Sylvia Plath's novel, a thinly disguised account of the poet's own descent into madness. The movie, on Channel 49, has been on for fifteen minutes, and shows the actress Marilyn Hassett, all high cheekbones and long silky blond hair, gracefully fending off the tentative lesbian advances of a friend.

Both Dawna and her sister watch, impassive. There's not much choice: the Smothers Brothers on Channel 2, a *Growing Pains* they've already seen on 6, *Aaron's Way* with some dumb blind musician on 8, that stupid Geraldo what's-his-name on Channel 12, and the short, smart-mouthed lady from *Cheers* going on and on about "the child-care problem" on Channel 10.

Second-Year Resident Jan Leigh comes into Room 16. Dawna and her sister abruptly stop talking. The only sound is Sylvia Plath talking with her lesbian friend.

"Let's turn the TV *off*," says Dr. Leigh. It is not a question, not even a suggestion. Snatching the remote from the hand of the laboring thirteen-year-old, the resident snaps the screen blank. "We don't need TV when the baby's being born!"

Grimly, the doctor examines the baby's heart tracings on the long skinny paper, then leaves the room, pulling it shut with an authoritative *whoosh!*

When a minute or so has passed, LaTreesha opens the door and looks down the hall to make sure Dr. Leigh is truly gone. Then she shakes her head, takes the remote control from the bedside table, and zaps the television set back on.

"*Sheesh!*" says LaTreesha. "She *one big bitch*! Huh, Dawna?"

Jan Leigh has a certain regal way of carrying herself, a don't-give-me-any-crap air. Nobody can say Jan Leigh hasn't done it herself, that she hasn't paid her dues.

However, this resident is white and she's middle class, and she suffers from the common delusion that television has little to do with "real life." Dr. Leigh mistakenly presumes that the immediacy of Dawna Hawkins's labor, the arrival of her child, is "real" to the girl, a child herself. That on some profound (perhaps even spiritual) level, this moment is realer to Dawna than the drawn-out, pretentious agonies of a poet the thirteen-year-old mother-to-be has most assuredly never read.

It may, of course, simply be that Second-Year Resident Jan Leigh is tired, in fact exhausted, by having just gotten married right smack in the middle of her residency. Her curtness may be explained by the fact that she's on the raggedy tail end of a thirty-six-hour shift. It may well be that Dr. Jan Leigh can't stand Sylvia Plath's poetry, never could understand why she would abandon two infant children by killing herself—if Dr. Leigh even happened to notice what was on the screen.

121

Dr. Jan Leigh has led a somewhat tumultuous life, with her share of sorrows and difficulties. God knows she's worked hard, plenty hard, to get where she is. In fact, it sometimes seems to her that it's all been one long series of odd jobs as she's scrabbled out a life for herself.

As a teenager, the daughter of two schoolteachers in sub-urban Detroit, Jan Leigh didn't get along with her parents. At twelve or so, when her mother returned to work, she was stuck with all the household chores, the cooking and cleaning and baby-sitting after school. Right after she finished high school (she had to wait that long or they swore they'd pack her off to a juvenile home), she took off in a van with a bunch of friends, headed for California and the hippie life. That was 1972. After a couple of years, she was living in a communal household in Santa Cruz, playing the piano, doing yoga and meditation, working as a part-time janitor to pay her $35 share of the monthly rent. She traveled to Mexico, worked in a California frozen food factory, doing the Brussels sprouts, the spinach, and all the rest. It was horrible, demeaning work. How could people do this seasonal labor all their working lives, returning year after year to stand there eight hours a day: one-two, one-two, one-two, just like a machine? She spent two years roaming around, doing odd jobs. Finally, she decided it was time to go back to school.

The University of California at Santa Cruz is one of those liberal no-grades progressive schools. It's set in the redwood forest, and you amble along idyllic paths from classroom to classroom. Jan thought maybe she'd be a bilingual education teacher, working with Hispanic high schoolers. She studied her butt off that first year, and did really well, top of her class in calculus and chemistry. And she met Dave, her first hus-band. Together, they went to Guatemala and lived with fam-ilies there, took a quarter off to work for the U.S. Forest Service. Went to Mexico. All through this, she'd been working at an ice cream store, working her way up from being just a server to counter manager, and finally to actually making the ice cream, which was fun.

Doing a tutorial at a high school, dodging spit wads and watching the kids pass notes all during class, Jan Leigh realized she did not want to be a high school teacher, after all. Too much police work.

She still wanted to speak Spanish, to work with people. Somehow Jan got the idea of being a nurse-practitioner. She didn't want to be a doctor, but she wanted to do more than a nurse does. She went to a junior college for a year, got the rest of her prerequisites out of the way.

She and Dave moved up to the Bay Area to help care for his mother, who was dying of cancer. Dave decided he wanted to be a doctor, and he went to UC Davis for pre-med courses. They commuted back and forth, Jan having gotten her nursing degree. After some six years of being together, the two finally married.

She had fallen in love with birthing and babies, and was working L&D at a small private hospital, focusing now on becoming a nurse-midwife. After a year, Jan figured she wasn't really cut out for nursing, wasn't even sure anymore about being a midwife. Present during a couple of real obstetrical nightmares, she realized that she couldn't honestly tell patients that, as a midwife, she could do everything a doctor could do. She had qualms about the 1 percent of deliveries that don't go well, didn't want to stand there wringing her hands waiting for a doctor to show up and do the c-section.

What to do? Finally, Jan Leigh had to face the truth: She was going to be a doctor. Dave was doing all the pre-med stuff, applying to med schools, and doing pretty well. But he was getting itchy feet, seeing other women on the side. They blew up, had big fights. Jan went through a huge depression, lost fifteen pounds in two weeks, totally fell apart. Dave got into med school at Irvine, and moved to Southern California. Jan was in Davis, doing pre-med, sending off applications. For months afterward, they waffled. Then Jan got into Irvine, too, and ended up there. Eventually, they divorced.

Though it was painful seeing her ex-husband around, Jan loved medical school, thrived on the academics. The first year, she worked as a nurse every other weekend, scheduling her hours when she didn't have a big test on Monday. It made for no free time, at all. But sixteen bucks an hour was pretty hard to pass up. After graduation, two years ago, with her classmate and roommate Kathleen Doyle, she came north to OHSU to check out the residency program. The two young women decided it was the program for them, the only one they saw that had any alternative birthing philosophy. OHSU seemed more humane and interested in the residents as people, with some balance of personal and professional life.

As it's turned out, the biggest problem is simply the fault of any OB/GYN residency program: You just can't work 80 to 110 hours a week and function well.

Best of all is Jan's new husband. Marc Gaudin is, oh happy day, not a doctor. He has a woodworking business. It's really nice, really refreshing, that his expertise is in areas Jan knows nothing about. He's good at business and investments. And he's into working out, and is willing to work out with her. Dave would never do that because he always said Jan was too slow for him. Marc and she met windsurfing, and at first Jan thought, *This guy's probably too nice for me. It's not going to work.* But he's so warm and giving. She's gotten used to it.

One of the things Marc did was make Jan sit down and tell him how much money she owed. It's all so depressing that she hadn't looked at it in ages. They added everything up yesterday, and she's $31,000 in the hole! That's in spite of all her many loans and scholarships—even one from the Daughters of the American Revolution!

For Dr. Leigh and many of the others working in L&D, it's an abiding mystery why a laboring woman of any age would want to watch television. They don't grasp that the picture on the screen may be richer, fuller—or at the very least no less real—than the picture of their own parched lives. Or that the noise and the flickering images simply make the women and their families feel comfortable, at home.

For Dawna Hawkins, the image on the TV screen above is neither realer, nor less real, than the first night Andy, her mother's live-in boyfriend, let himself into a ten-year-old's sleeping nest on the couch, shoving her Cabbage Patch doll out of the way, and helping himself to what the slumbering, already developed child had to offer. The way Andy looked at it, access to her big-titty daughters was part of what he had coming to him for living with that stupid fat bitch.

And the baby coming three months ahead of schedule?

That's no more real to Dawna Hawkins than the cartoons she watches on Saturday mornings.

Nothing in the sixth-grader's life has changed much because of being pregnant. It isn't going to keep her from finishing high school, because Dawna's just waiting until she can drop out, anyway. Being big and fat with the baby hasn't kept Andy from poking his thing into her three or four times a week, still. (One night when he was really drunk, he brought home three of his drinking buddies, and let them put their things in her, too. One of them really hurt her, because he put his thing in the other hole, but her mother still didn't stop them, just stood in the corner watching, and Andy just kept laughing and laughing.)

It would never occur to Dawna to complain, to believe that her mother had a responsibility to protect her, any more than it will occur to her, a decade from now, to protect the daughter she's giving birth to tonight.

Her sister knows all about it. At twenty, LaTreesha already has three children. Her first, from a rape when she was eleven, when she was just walking home from school. The second was from Andy. This last one, at least, is from her own boyfriend, so things are getting better.

2121: 9:21 P.M.

Because of all the tiny, premature, and low-birth-weight babies expected in the next few hours, several staff neonatologists, on call but at home, have been summoned to come in tonight.

In Room 2, Patti Rausch, still wearing her tan-red-and-green argyle socks, pushes out an 8-pound, 2½-ounce girl named Tami Rae. After a swift examination by the nurse-midwife, the newborn is whisked down and across the hall to the nursery.

"Is she okay?" asks the father, following the nurse. His baseball cap, with NW ENVIRONCON stitched on it, is twisted in his hands. "Is she okay?"

"Oh, yeah." Nurse Carolyn Bachhuber smiles. "She just wasn't pinking up as fast as we like."

125

Relieved, pulling his cap back onto his head, Tami Rae Rausch's father returns to Room 2 and the mother of his three children. He kisses her soundly on both cheeks.

"Honey, when you're feeling up to it, I think we'd better go out and buy us some more of them lucky socks," says Jeffrey Rausch, eyebrows waggling under the baseball cap.

"Oh, Jeffie!" says his wife, laughing and crying at once.

2217: 10:17 P.M.

In Room 16, Dawna Hawkins has a big contraction. The thirteen-year-old makes a noise that begins as a moan and ends as a scream. On the TV screen above, the willowy blond poet, who has been committed to a fancy mental hospital, has just discovered her lesbian friend dead, swinging from a rope. LaTreesha, twenty-year-old mother of three, holds her little sister's foot, squeezing the toes with her fingers, keeping her eye on the drama on the screen above.

The sisters are not the lone witnesses of the trials of Sylvia Plath. There's Nurse Carolyn Bachhuber, and freckly Nurse Mary from the Intermediate Neonatal Care Unit. There's also a nurse-midwifery student and a medical student. First-Year Resident Linda Moore, who is black, is delivering the premature baby. She has left the television on.

Finally, at 2224, 10:24 P.M., a little girl is born, weighing 1,340 grams, just under three pounds. Three months behind the normal gestation time of forty weeks, the tiny infant looks like a newly hatched bird, with barely discernible nipples.

On the television set above, the poet, aided by her motherly psychiatrist, has "come to terms" with the hanging suicide of her lesbian friend, according to the actress's voice-over narration concluding the movie:

> To the person in the bell jar, blank and stopped as a
> dead baby, the world itself is the bad dream. I asked
> her if I would survive. She said, "Yes." And with that,
> she at once freed me and condemned me back to life.
> If I am the arrow, I cannot fly through darkness.

CHAPTER NINE

DAY 4: Thursday, April 14

("It's a chick!" exults the grandfather, one eye on the television screen.)

1535: 3:35 P.M.

THE WORD HAS SIFTED down that Melody Richards has changed her mind. She's going to take her baby home with her. The blond eighteen-year-old will not, she now says from her bed in South Hospital, give her baby away to the Mormon couple from Utah. No way. Forget it. They can just *shove* their brand-new house with its teddy bear-filled nursery. Someone has been bringing the baby over from 4NE for Melody to nurse.

Melody feels her son's eager, sucking mouth on her breast, and she closes her eyes and thinks: *This is mine! This belongs to me! Nobody can take this away from me! This is Bradley Michael Richards and he is my son and he is mine mine mine mine mine!* She wonders how she could have even considered not being part of his everyday life. (She also wonders how she is going to get off welfare, how she can finish high school and get some more education. But she'll just think about that *later.*)

On hearing the news, Tracey Delaplain, the pregnant, Catholic resident who handed Melody her son right after delivering him, makes the clenched-fist power-to-the-people salute: *"Yeaaaay!"* Nurse Molly Wilson is less sanguine about this turn of events: She has two children, one adopted, the other born to her.

"You don't know," she tells Tracey, shaking her head slowly. "You just don't know."

Across town, in a ranch-style house on La Mancha Circle in the suburb of Tigard, Jack Bidwell comforts the weeping Mary Fran, who keeps telling him she feels like she's gone through a strenuous, agonizing labor, to finally hold a baby born silent and still. Hanging heavy in the air is the lush smell of the standing rib roast their cousin has been cooking for their planned celebration dinner.

"Doesn't it ever stop raining here?" asks Mary Fran, looking out the picture window at a huge blooming purple rhododendron, shining and dripping.

"Oh, yes," replies her cousin Sue, standing in the doorway between kitchen and living room. Awkwardly, she smooths out her apron. "Later in the spring." Mary Fran's cousin (who grew up with her, close as sisters, in Utah) has been crying, too, alone in the master bathroom.

"It's real pretty here in the summer," she offers.

"I just don't see how you can stand all this rain," says Mary Fran, turning back to her husband.

"Oh, Jack! Our baby! Our little Danny's *gone!*"

Jack Bidwell, whose throat feels tight and raw, just holds his wife and lets her cry.

Back up on Marquam Hill, on the fourth floor of an old brick building, hospital smells mingle with the aroma of freshly brewed coffee in the small room around the corner from the nurses' station. With The Board showing all L&D rooms filled, there is little time to debate Melody's change of heart.

In PAR is Melissa Shinkle, twenty-two years old and thirty-nine weeks along with her second child.

In Room 18, Renee Overmeyer is lying in her bed, wondering if they're going to have to give her a cesarean section, after all. She's twenty-one, a couple of weeks short of her due date, and the cute doctor with the moustache and the cleft chin told her she has what's called an "abruption." Something about the placenta coming loose where it shouldn't.

This lying and waiting isn't something a girl should have to do alone. When will she learn that sleeping with someone doesn't mean you have a "relationship" with him? At times with Bobby, it was sort of like they were playing parts in two completely separate movies. Only his movie has him off God-knows-where right now. "Thinking things over," says Bobby. *Thinking things over?* Terrific. Oh, well, Mom and Elise should show up pretty soon.

In Room 16, private nurse-midwifery patient Peggy Ames roosts in a rocking chair, rocking—*back*-forth, *back*-forth, *back*-forth—the chair making a soothing sort of creak on the forth part. Her husband, Ted, sits in an armchair pulled right up next to her and holds her hand. Ted Ames is ecstatic: The ultrasound taken a couple of hours ago revealed that the couple is, after two daughters, about to have a son.

"Anything I can do for you, honey?" Ted keeps asking.

A pleased, plump hen on her nest, his wife just smiles and shakes her head.

"Later, honey," she tells him. "I'm going to need your help later. Just ease up for now. Go get yourself a cup of coffee or something."

In Room 10, a thirty-six-year-old primigravida named Jill Yost pulls on what she calls her fat-preggie-girl pants and prepares to go home. Another false alarm, they told her, but it shouldn't be much longer. Having spent what feels like years of her life in aerobics classes, she is ready to get this baby out of her body, and her body straight back into her cute clothes. (She is quite determined she will stay a size seven, baby or no baby!)

The Board says that Wendy Bovey, in Room 8, is seventeen, HIV positive, and about to give birth to her second child. She hopes this one isn't going to be a little ratfuck like her sixteen-month-old. The nerve of the doctors telling her that the reason Jason is so cranky and never wants to be held may be because of the coke Wendy snorted when she was pregnant with him. Christ. She even stopped using a couple weeks before he was born, just to be safe, like the other girls told her to.

129

Wendy's been in here since nine this morning, and every fucking time she wants a cigarette, she has to traipse all the way down the fucking hall and down the fucking elevator to the fucking outside by the fucking garbage cans. As if she didn't feel like barfing already! You'd think they'd have a little more *courtesy* for the patients around here! After all, our tax dollars pay their salaries. They work for us. Not that Wendy Bovey has paid any taxes in her life. What's she going to put down for "occupation" on the tax form: "I have my very own corner on Union Avenue"? Well, Wendy sure has an honest answer ready for the NAME OF FATHER blank on this kid's birth certificate: UNKNOWN.

In the Exam Room, Suzanne Wilson has been brought up from the Mother-Baby Unit on 3NW for monitoring. Twenty-one-year-old Suzanne, who's been in the MBU since late last night, has been complaining of pain that seems unduly severe for such an early stage of labor. She wants them to give her something. They don't want to.

Suzanne has never been much of a one for pain. When she has a headache, she takes a Valium. When she's depressed, she has a drink. And if she's still depressed, she smokes a joint. This is *real pain*, goddammit, and she wants something for it.

"I'll talk with a doctor and let you know what we can do," says a nurse. "Try to relax." She hands Suzanne the remote for the television set.

Nurse Sharon Menasche, everyone agrees, is very good with Room 2's Darleen Robinson, an FLM—Funny-Looking Mom—and then some.

In the room at this moment, along with the nurse, are FLM Darleen, her husband, Joe, and her mother. According to her chart and nurses' station scuttlebutt, Darleen has some kind of seizure disorder. Just what sort is unspecified and evidently undiagnosed, but the result is a highly unpleasant twenty-two-year-old primigravida, her usually childish behavior exacerbated by her labor. Weighing probably 275 pounds, a furious Darleen sits up in her bed.

"What's going *on* here?" she asks. "What's going *on* here?"

Darleen's husband sits in a chair in front of the window, PORTLAND TRAIL BLAZERS baseball cap pulled forward over

130

frizzy gold hair, plaid flannel shirt rolled up above the elbows, showing a self-inflicted tattoo of a cross on his right forearm. Through dark-rimmed glasses, he glances in apparent unconcern at his laboring wife. Darleen's mother, a gaunt woman of sixty-five or thereabouts, her thin white hair pinned severely to the top of her head, rocks in the chair at the end of the room. Every two or three minutes, she looks up from her copy of *The Plain Truth,* its cover boasting row upon row of white grave-marker crosses. She glares, purse-lipped, at her distraught daughter.

On the television set, turned on but ignored, the cast of *thirtysomething* visits Phil Donahue. An earnest red-bearded actor whines that strangers in supermarkets mistake him for the insensitive twit he portrays on the popular series.

When the nurse has Darleen turn her back, the open gown reveals a dozen or so freshly squeezed pimples. With short, stubby fingers, their metallic red polish nearly all chewed off, Darlene worries the zits on her fleshy face.

Dr. Terry Jones, anesthesiology resident, enters the room, announcing he's here to help Darleen with the pain. She is in midcontraction.

"It *hurts* me," she screams. *"Get rid of it! Get rid of it!"*

Dr. Jones is laid-back—the Quickest Epidural in the West, according to the L&D nurses—and with his very own pregnant wife at home. He explains mildly that what he's about to do will get rid of the pain.

Darleen takes one look at the needle that this strange man wants to plunge into her back and screams: *"Ma-maaaaaaaa!"*

Her mother looks up from her religious tract for five seconds, max, then returns to her reading and rocking.

"Ready to have that pain go away?" asks Nurse Sharon.

"Please make it go away! I'm scared!"

Dr. Jones preps Darleen's back with Betadine, readying it for the epidural line that will go into her spinal column.

"Ow-*eee*!" she shrieks, like a preschooler who's just jumped into a cold swimming pool. "He must like to give women goose bumps—especially me! Is he a doctor?"

Through all this, Nurse Sharon Menasche stands by Darleen's side, her hand tenderly rubbing the patient's shoulder as Dr. Jones deftly threads the epidural into the patient's back.

131

With astonishing swiftness, the anesthesia seizes control of Darleen's body.

"My *legs*!" she shrieks, panic on the pimpled face. "Where are they? Where's my *legs*? Where are they? I can't feel them!"

The nurse pulls the sheet aside, showing Darleen that her stubble-haired legs are still there, pink-painted toenails and all.

"Why do you have four eyes?" she asks the nurse.

"Why do you have two heads?" she asks the anesthesiology resident. Her eyes narrow against the vile plot against her.

"You'll be fine now," says Dr. Jones, giving her shoulder a pat as he exits Room 2.

The silent old woman keeps on rocking, while on the unwatched TV screen, impassioned Donahue audience members grill the red-bearded actor who portrays a glib advertising man.

1656: 4:56 P.M.

At the nurses' station, Third-Year Resident Julie Bouchard, her stomach still feeling odd, is on the phone telling someone that patients are being sent over to North Portland's Emanuel Hospital. (Tuesday night's romp with Glenn in the sleeping room upstairs couldn't have made her feel queasy *this* early, could it?)

"All our patients on The Board are in active labor and can't be moved," says the slender, dark-haired resident. (Maybe some soda crackers? Tea?)

Dr. Kirk tells Julie that Dr. Amanda Clark is trying to find out how many laboring women Emanuel can accept.

"We need to log how many we send there, so the others can be sent to Good Sam," says the department chairman.

A few feet away from the department chairman and the resident, Marisa Johnsrud slumps in a wheelchair, new blue terry robe tied around her old yellow flannel granny gown with pink rosebuds. One of Dr. Kirk's private patients, Marisa is miserable, near tears as she studies the huge lesions on her fingers.

Marisa is unmarried, her boyfriend dumped her two

months into her pregnancy, and—given all the time off she's had to take in the last few months—she's pretty sure she's about to be fired from her job as an insurance adjuster. But right now, none of this matters. What matters is that she wants, more than anything in the world, to have this baby turn out okay.

Marisa Johnsrud has lupus, which is threatening the life of her thirty-four-week-old fetus. With Marisa's kind of systemic lupus, an inflammatory connective-tissue disorder which in her case has invaded her body well beyond the obvious skin manifestations, there are a lot of pregnancy losses. The masses of medications necessary to save her life, combined with her malfunctioning kidneys, haven't done much for Marisa's baby. As suspected, and confirmed by the ultrasound, the fetus is growth-retarded, with no gross body movements and decreased amniotic fluid.

All considered, the low BPP, biophysical profile, has led to the decision to perform a cesarean section on Marisa Johnsrud tonight.

One of a group of diseases called "collagen vascular diseases," lupus primarily affects the body tissues made up of collagen, a form of protein found in tissues, and the blood vessels that make them elastic. Collagen vascular diseases are thought to be immunological in nature, resulting from abnormalities of the immune system. They are also believed to be inflammatory diseases.

There is no question that sometimes pregnancy is a risk factor for a lupus flare, or relapse. Lupus itself seems the most common collagen vascular disease compromising pregnancy, occurring in about one in 1,500 to 3,000 deliveries. If a woman has had severe lupus, if there's evidence of kidney failure, often it's impossible for her to become pregnant. If she does become pregnant, she may have great difficulty carrying the pregnancy.

Sitting in her wheelchair across from the nurses' station, fingering the sleeve of her old flannel nightgown, Marisa Johnsrud shows the classic signs of lupus. There's a rash across her face, in the classic "butterfly" distribution, across her nose and down the cheeks. She has angry red disclike lesions on her skin. Marisa also has an arthritis-like inflammation of the lining of her body cavities, and of the linings around her heart and lungs. Her kidneys have been excreting protein that can't be reabsorbed. Mercifully, she has escaped the seizures and psychoses that often accompany a lupus flare.

Lupus in a pregnant woman is very bad for the baby, with early pregnancy loss—miscarriages or spontaneous abortions—possibly as high as 90 percent. Clinically recognized miscarriage from lupus may be as high as 30 percent. Once a pregnancy is established, the effects on the fetus depend to some extent on the severity of the disease. A woman who suffers a severe lupus relapse at any point in her pregnancy may have only a 50 percent to 65 percent chance of delivering a live baby. If the lupus has been complicated by severe kidney disease, or there is evidence of kidney failure, lower those chances to 50 percent or less.

The hapless baby's in utero suffering may or may not be due to the lupus itself. The mother may have undergone intensive medical therapy, and the powerful drugs may certainly affect the fetus. The placenta itself—the very source of the baby's nourishment and continued life—may be badly damaged by the inflammation or by damage to the mother's heart and kidneys. Interuterine growth retardation may result. Further, there is such a thing as neonatal lupus syndrome: An infant may be born with manifestations of the disease, presumably because the mother's abnormal antibodies have crossed over the placenta to the fetus. The infant may have heart and blood abnormalities or severe anemia from the breakdown of red blood cells. Additionally, there may be a congenital heart block, in which the small human being's heart rate is uncontrolled by its natural pacemaker. Death from this may be as high as 30 percent. However, even with neonatal lupus syndrome, without heart-block complications the prognosis tends to be good, the signs becoming resolved by the baby's first birthday.

With Marisa Johnsrud, the decision was made to hospitalize her and start her on a daily regimen of 100 to 200 milligrams of the steroid Prednisone given intravenously, in order to improve her clinical response. It was important to increase her platelet count, to improve her kidney function, and to resolve her bleeding.

Marisa Johnsrud did not improve quickly, and she was put on azathiaprine and cyclophosphamide, both very powerful cytotoxic drugs meant specifically to kill dividing cells. It was important to partially knock out Marisa's immune system, almost as though she had severe leukemia, since it was sending abnormal, harmful antibodies that were trying to destroy her body. Then, the effects of the medications were closely followed with laboratory tests. Often twice daily, the doctors looked at Marisa's complete blood count: platelets, kidney function, electrolytes, sodium, potassium, chloride, liver count, antibodies.

All along, as had been done since it was determined that Marisa Johnsrud had a viable pregnancy, the series of ultrasounds continued, with an eye for evidence of severe growth retardation. The estimated fetal weights were noted and recorded. With a cardiac echo, the fetal heart was looked at, to determine if heart block had developed. It was important, too, to see if Marisa's baby had heart failure coming on, if the fetus had started to swell up, sequestering fluid in its tissues.

All of these procedures, of course, were done in consultation with hematologists, nephrologists, kidney specialists, cardiologists, and rheumatologists.

Dozens of tests. Endless visits. Shots. Medicines that make her throw up. And here she is, a frightened and very sick thirty-two-year-old woman, thirty-six weeks into an awful pregnancy, sitting in a wheelchair on Pill Hill's 4NE, waiting. Waiting to find out what's going to happen. Waiting to find out whether she will, when it's all over, have a darling little child to take home and love.

In the coffee/supply room, the residents compete for who gets to section Victoria Sanchez, who is having twins. (Why? Because it's *fun*.)

The winners are Julie Bouchard and Second-Year Resident Brian Clark. Dr. Amanda Clark will be the staff doctor overseeing the work of the two residents.

In OR 2, seventeen-year-old Victoria and her husband, Manuel, are being prepared for the surgery as Dr. Mandy Clark ambles in. She explains to the couple that their babies must be delivered this way because they are in the breech position. Manuel, eager dark eyes shining from his pock-marked face behind the blue paper mask, is asking what happens to the babies right away when they're out.

"The first baby will be kept right here," explains Pediatrics Fellow Don Buffkin. "The second one will be taken to an identical setup right in the hall outside."

1753: 5:53 P.M.

A boy is out, and handed straight to Dr. Buffkin and the nurse and medical students. Then, a girl! Together, the twins add up to 5,785 grams—the little boy weighing 6.8 pounds, and his sister, 5.9 pounds. In the hall outside, the little girl (who has long, slender fingers like her father) doesn't have good color or aspirations—her Apgar score is only 4—and she is taken into the Intermediate Neonatal Care Unit down the hall. The boy's Apgar is an 8 or 9.

1800: 6 P.M.

Darleen Robinson, the "seizure disorder" in Room 2, may end up having to be sectioned, the assembly of students, nurses, residents, and staff is told during Board Rounds.

Unit Secretary Jaynee Bounseville, usually on the night shift, is working the earlier shift this evening. Looking up from the big box of Dunkin' Donuts she's brought in for the sugar-junkie crew, she says she was working one night when Darleen came in a couple of weeks back.

"'I had a seizure!' she kept saying," reports Jaynee, a vibrant, funny, dark-haired, *zaftig* woman of thirty or so. "And when they did the ultrasound, she said to her husband: 'Look, honey—it's still an *egg*!'"

Jaynee shakes her head, taking another slurp of coffee between bites of jelly-filled doughnut.

"My kid, *she* knows where babies come from," says Jaynee, laughing. "She's four, you know? She says to me, 'You just put a quarter in your belly button, and you *push* and *push* and *push* real hard for a long time, and the baby pops out! And then you just *cut the quarter!*' "

There is laughter for this.

"And when I asked her who told her that, she just says, 'I just knew it in my *brain,* Mom!' "

1855: 6:55 P.M.

Down in the Mother-Baby Unit, Hilary Blanchard can finish only half of the dessert delivered with her dinner from Briggs & Crampton. It looked good, but it was simply too much on top of the rest: huge prawns sautéed with butter and white wine and just a little bit of shallot; a pretty green salad with simple vinaigrette dressing and garnished with edible tulip petals. And the catering service's famous toasted hazelnut-rye bread. The dessert was early spring strawberries, along with cut-up pieces of tropical fruit—pineapple, kiwi, and papaya, all nestled into a bowl with the season's first tender little shoots of fresh mint.

Hilary picks up her needlepoint, spreading it across the tops of her legs, raised under the covers. But before threading the yarn through the canvas, she rings the bell alongside her bed. No sense wasting the dessert. Maybe the nurses would like to finish it up.

1949: 7:49 P.M.

It's about ten to eight, and the windows of the coffee/supply room let in the soft, gathering dusk as preparations are being made to section Marisa Johnsrud, the woman with lupus. The contrast with the anticipated c-section delivery of the Sanchez twins less than two hours ago is dramatic. Then, the residents were practically flipping a coin to see who got to unzip the teenaged Victoria Sanchez's belly and take out her babies.

The difference in the anticipated cesarean section is not that, unlike Victoria Sanchez, Marisa Johnsrud is a private patient. It's that Marisa is very sick, and her baby is not necessarily going to live. Everything is handled without any of the usual stress-reducing banter. Instead, there is a quiet, near-religious solemnity. The surgery will be headed up by Second-Year Resident Brian Clark and Staff Doctor Amanda Clark. They are unrelated, but in jollier moments are known as "The Clark Twins."

At 8:33, in OR2 the doctors deliver Marisa Johnsrud's tiny daughter. While everyone in the room, except for Marisa, is wearing a paper face mask covering all but eyes and a bit of forehead, the strain and worry are obvious. Marisa's premature baby weighs only 3¾ pounds. She is solemnly cleaned up by Pediatrics Fellow Don Buffkin, stationed at the side of the operating room.

He judges the Apgar to be an 8, surprisingly good. The tiny infant, in her little pink-and-white striped knit cap, is swaddled in warm receiving blankets printed with pastel bunnies and ducks, and swiftly transported down the hall to INCU.

Behind the curtain, sparing Marisa Johnsrud from the sight of her pale green, blood-drenched surgical draperies, tears course down the cheeks of a woman just delivered of her first and undoubtedly only child.

2134: 9:34 P.M.

Alison Gill, who has been in labor since eight last night, and who checked into Pill Hill at noon, is oh, so tired of pushing. In the Special Delivery Room with her is just about every member of her family, dutifully assembled for the spectator sport that a birthing has become. There's her mother, thin and nervous, with a short blond bob. Her mother's friend Francie, who's along for the ride, having known eighteen-year-old Alison since she and her twin sister were in kindergarten. Alison's father, divorced for years from her mother, has a three-year-old and a six-month-old back home in Beaverton with his current "lady." Alison's stepfather is expected to make an appearance momentarily, and his arrival is eagerly anticipated. (Hey, he's the only one who knows how to work the video camera!)

Alison's twin sister Jasmine (née Charlene) lurks sulkily

138

in the corner of the Special Delivery Room, nervously running her $45 porcelain fingernails through bleached, waistlong tresses. Whenever someone new enters the room, the reed-thin teenager, in the Guess? jeans (so tight she has to lie down to zip them) informs the newcomer that she and Alison are twins.

"You'd never *guess* we were twins, would you?" asks Jasmine/Charlene, hope shining through the querulous voice. "I mean, with her being so *heavy* and having that brown *hair,* you wouldn't even *think* we were *sisters,* would you?" Ignored by staff and visitor alike, she goes back to threading carmine-tipped fingers through her hair. Fishing a mirror from her bag, she peers intently at her eyes, one long fingernail flicking a chunk of caked mascara from a rouged cheek.

"You're doing good, Alison—super!" says Nurse Barbara Stoutenberg.

"Thanks," says the pretty young pregnant woman on the bed, reaching up to shift the folded wet white washcloth on her forehead.

Her bearded, handsome father, who is holding Alison's right hand, leans down to give her a hug and a kiss. Straightening up, he returns his gaze to the television screen, which shows the Portland Trail Blazers in hot contest with the Utah Jazz.

"Ooooh, Kiki!" he bellows to the image of Trail Blazer Kiki Vandeweghe. Back to Alison: *"Push,* angel . . . *push,* sweetie!" Again, to the television set, he intones: "They're only two points ahead . . . ten seconds left in the game!"

"Okay, Alison, take a deep breath," instructs the nurse.

Between contractions, the atmosphere in the room eases briefly.

" . . . and I'm never having kids!" says Jasmine/Charlene in the corner, muttering to nobody in particular.

"Alison always said she was going to adopt Korean kids," says the grandmother-to-be. "Yin and Yang Gill!"

Resident Gary Hoffman enters the room for the delivery. Handsome and relaxed, he piques the interest of Jasmine/Charlene, who smooths her jeans over her round little rump, venturing closer to the birthing bed to investigate this intriguing new development.

"Hi!" she says breathily, tossing back the glittering mane.

"Hi," the resident replies.

Alison has another contraction, a big one this time. She pushes, hard.

"Atta girl!" says Gary Hoffman.

"Good girl...*super*, Alison!" says Barb Stoutenberg.

"Push that baby *outta* there, Alison!" says her father.

Gary Hoffman leaves the room to bring in some solutions needed for the final part of the delivery.

"Dad?" says Alison.

"Yeah, baby?"

"Dad, be on this side," she says.

As Dr. Hoffman reenters Special Delivery, Alison's tall, husky father obeys his laboring daughter, joining his former wife on Alison's left side. The once-married couple exchange a look of warmth, and they reel against one another, a stilted substitute for a hug.

"Did you call Tom?" the father asks Jasmine/Charlene.

"Yeah, I *called* Tom!" is the sullen reply.

Just then, Tom makes his entrance, and father and step-father sort of bump together in awkward male greeting. The stepfather can't work the video camera, either. Oh, well.

"That's okay, you guys—don't worry about it," says Alison. "I want to push! I really want to *p-u-u-u-sh*!" She lets out a noise that's halfway between a scream and a laugh.

"Doing great, Alison! Doing just great!" says Dr. Gary Hoffman.

As the baby comes out, all the spectators—even Jasmine/Charlene—lean forward to see the important detail.

"It's a *chick*!" exults the new grandfather, Alison's father.

The "chick," weighing 8½ pounds, is named Amanda Jayne.

A short, plump woman, sister of the laboring Peggy Ames, bustles agitatedly out of Room 16 and over to the nurses' station.

"Water," she says breathlessly. "Where can I get a glass of water?"

"Well, she can't have water at this stage of her labor," replies a nurse, not unkindly. "Maybe some ice."

"No, no! It's not for her. It's for me. I'm on Weight Watchers, and I haven't had my six to eight glasses of water today!"

The nurse points her to the little room outside the bathroom.

"There's paper cups and water in there," she says, smiling.

In the coffee/supply room, three residents, a nurse, and a medical student spoon Rocky Road ice cream into Styrofoam coffee cups, digging into the half-gallon someone just brought in from the convenience store a little way up the hill.

"Ambrosia!" exclaims one, sucking like a nursing infant on a white plastic spoon. "Pure ambrosia!"

"Sugar," replies another. "Pure sugar!"

Seven miles away, in a North Portland bedroom with an empty crib, Harriet Grackle sits in a position as nearly cross-legged as her belly will allow. Her calves are numb, and have been for the past half hour. Pretty soon, she's going to have to pee, and she'll just have to ask for help getting up.

Biting her lower lip in concentration, Harriet paints a chest of drawers she got for $5.00 at a thrift shop this afternoon. The chest is the perfect height for diaper-changing, and using bits of leftover enamel, she's devised a plot. The basic shell will be a royal blue, and each drawer will be a different bright color. So far tonight, one drawer's been painted yellow, one red and one purple. There's only the green one to go.

"Harriet? Honey?" Animal Grackle stands in the doorway to the nursery. "I can't help thinking that paint stink is bad for you."

"Almost done, Animal. Isn't it pretty?"

Her husband smiles at her. How on earth, he wonders for the millionth time, did he get such a smart, beautiful woman to marry him and have his kid?

2324: 11:24 P.M.

Outside the northwest wing of the hospital, two women stand and smoke cigarettes, trying to keep from getting soaked in the April rain polishing the parking lot's darkly brilliant rhododendron bushes. Exhausted and drained by her daughter's sixteen-hour ordeal, Alison Gill's mother tells her friend that the worst part was when, there for a while, they thought they might have to cut Alison open to get the baby out safely.

"Yeah," says her friend, taking a deep, satisfying drag on her Virginia Slims. "Me, too. I could tell it was getting to you." The cool rain splashes on her red-framed glasses, parting her long dark brown hair into matted dreadlocks.

"Yin and Yang Gill?" she asks, shaking her head. "Come on, did Alison *really* say that? You made that up!"

The two women laugh, more than the little joke deserves.

CHAPTER TEN

DAY 5: Friday, April 15

(Lily Pratt becomes a mother.)

1552: 3:52 P.M.

EXCEPT FOR HER HUSBAND, nobody knows that 468-pound Lily Pratt's main fear is that she will make a lot of awful, embarrassing noises while the baby is coming. Down in the Mother-Baby Unit, she's been hearing all those moans and screams from the other women before they're transported upstairs to 4NE. And if there's anything this large woman hates, it's making a spectacle of herself, more so than her size already does. For all of her life, Lily has yearned to be delicate and tasteful. Ladylike.

On this damp Friday, the skies above Pill Hill unusually smoggy, Lily's son is going to make his exit from his mother's body. Lily has endeared herself to the staff and residents in her days in the hospital. She makes no special requests, appreciating everything done for her, taking the trouble to learn the names of the nurses and residents who come into her room. She has been kind and interested in the half dozen women who have shared her room in the Mother-Baby Unit. Even though there's still an occasional titter at her weight during

Board Rounds, the shared and sincere hope is that Lily Pratt will not have to be sectioned.

Throughout the previous night, Lily was constantly "taken to the back," transported into one of the emergency rooms as the residents on 4NE feared that they were going to have to get the baby out by cesarean section, after all. Her baby's heart tracing was poor, and there was an abiding fear that at the estimated ten or eleven pounds, Lily's child would not fare well through a vaginal delivery. While the staff likes Lily— loves her, in fact, for her beautiful personality—the worry and the fright of the impending, ghastly cesarean section, often gets translated into a gallows, *M*A*S*H*-like humor. In a similar case, an obese woman died last year over at Bess Kaiser from c-section complications.

Second-Year Resident Karen Hill, pushing forty, is weary of what she views as all the crummy sexist jokes about Lily's size. And angry. She's glad she's the one who'll deliver this baby.

Karen Hill is a straightforward, shortish, squarish woman, a mother of two teenagers, who finds this adolescent Mickey Mouse crap hard to take. Some of the male residents and medical students seem so loftily amused, almost personally *offended,* by Lily's obesity. Standing around during Board Rounds, they giggle like junior high schoolers.

Okay, if they have to give Lily a c-section, it's going to be difficult. The plan is to try for a regular vaginal birth, but they just might have to do an emergency section. And in that case, you have to skip a lot of steps, and with her size, there'd be so much retraction, pulling back all that fat. But what we're talking about here is a *surgical problem,* and the frustration with the potential difficulties gets automatically translated into a denigration of the woman herself. Instead of stating the simple fact—*this is a large, obese woman*—they do all the emotional-content things that our culture does to large women. Board-Rounds snickering still invades the profession. The old standards of evaluating the patient on thinness is just a spinout of how our society defines physical attractiveness. It's just wrong for surgeons to blame the patient for the difficulty of the surgery itself. And, oh, they do!

Dr. Karen Hill has the fear that patients are going to overhear some of the cracks made by residents. They're so judgmental. Her own judgmentalness bothers Karen. It's the drug-abusing patients who test *her* tolerance level. From the time she was a first-year resident, an intern, Karen believes she's seeing at least five times as many drug abusers on 4NE. That's just one year, and just the women who either admit it or act so peculiar that they get screened for drug use. Or the babies get screened. You don't need the mother's permission to screen a baby once it's born. Sometimes you just have to do it. You have to know what the newborns are withdrawing from, to figure out how to treat them.

One time a woman came into the prep room. Using IV crack on a frequent basis, she told them. Karen gave her an ultrasound and saw that the baby was turning somersaults in the uterus. Literally. Right there on the screen, like on a television set, you could see the limbs jerking and kicking, the baby shifting from being all over on the left side of the woman's abdomen to being on the right side. That baby was so stimulated by the crack that it would change from breech to vertex several times in the space of a few minutes. Watching this, knowing that that fetus was in agony in the very place where it should have been safe, Dr. Karen Hill became physically sick, knew she had to leave the room.

Yet, looking at the woman, the resident could tell that she was an addict, and out of control. That she needed treatment like anyone else. The woman with the baby relentlessly spinning in her womb wasn't oriented in time or place, didn't even know where she was. Looking at her chart, Karen discovered that the woman had suffered a horrible childhood herself: sexual abuse, physical abuse, alcoholic parents. She hadn't come to be this way by choice. There was enough pain to go around in this one.

1610: 4:10 P.M.

The Board shows that, as usual, all of L&D's rooms are full. Lily Pratt is awaiting the next stage in Room 10.

In PAR is Brenda Sommers, a private patient whose labor

is so slow and unadvanced that she will be sent home late tonight.

In Room 18 is Karla Michaels, twenty-two, who has been sent to The Hill from Tillamook, on the Oregon coast, because of problems with her labor.

In Room 16, Carmen Ramirez, a tiny woman of twenty-two, is being soothed in Spanish by Nurse Jeanne Gates. Her husband, Pablo, as befits a Hispanic husband, sits in a straight chair right outside the door, awaiting the arrival of his first-born.

In Room 8, Joni Phillips glares at her timid, dark husband. A small and sour-tempered woman of twenty-nine, with asthma and an accelerated heart rate probably due to medication, Joni has a huge dark birthmark, raised and hairy, on the right side of her belly, midway between navel and crotch. She is having her third baby.

In the Exam Room, Betsy McDonald, a week short of her due date, is being told that she will probably be staying for the afternoon and evening, and leaving tomorrow with a baby. In the bed next to Betsy's, Gretchen Fisher, a wispy redhead with probably a month to go before her real labor begins, is being told to get ready to go home.

In Room 2, Clarice Morgan, sent to The Hill all the way from the coastal town of Newport, Oregon, is being transported downstairs to the Mother-Baby Unit. She's in labor, all right. But it's going to be a while before she pops.

Over in South Hospital, Melody Richards has changed her mind, again. After a long talk with the hospital social worker, the eighteen-year-old has decided she'll let the couple from Utah take her baby away with them on the train, after all. No, she assures the social worker, she won't change her mind again. It was just, well, seeing him and holding him and nursing him and all that, it just gave her these feelings that she wasn't expecting, that nobody told her she'd have.

Maybe someday, after she's finished high school, and gone to college even, and gotten a good job, she'll meet someone and get married and have some more children. And maybe someday, way in the future, she'll get to see her son, when he's like eighteen. And she'll tell him lots of things then. She'll tell him how hard it was to give him away to other people, how hard it was to have him vanish from her sight, from her life, probably forever. How hard it was to trust that he'd have a good life without his real mother to watch over him. And that it didn't mean she didn't love him or anything like that.

But there's this thing that keeps running through her head, like some dumb song you hear on the radio and it won't leave. (*Good-bye, good-bye, good-bye, my love . . . good-bye, good-bye, good-bye, my love . . . good-bye, good-bye, good-bye, my love . . .*)

Melody just wishes it would go away, and that she could stop crying.

On 4NE a nurse in the INCU evening shift asks a just-leaving day-shift nurse about the people who collected Melody's son this morning.

"What did they look like, the couple that took him away?"

"Blond," says the day-shift nurse. "Both of them, blond. Healthy. Mormon."

The nurse turns away quickly, awkwardly, so that the evening-shift nurse won't see the tears in her eyes. As she walks away from the nursery, her rubber-soled shoes (new that day) squeak, a small mournful cry unheard in a roomful of wailing feeders and growers, the mewling preemies in their warmers.

1625: 4:25 P.M.

Lily Pratt, in active labor, has been shifted into OR2 so that she can be swiftly prepared for a cesarean section if necessary. She wears a vast nightie of pink cotton plissé, printed with rosebuds of a darker pink. Covering her lower face is an oxygen mask of rigid green plastic. Her husband, David, drabbed out in green scrubs, paper booties and hair covering, and a blue paper face mask, holds her hand.

Nurse Becky Abramson bustles at the side of the room, checking a cabinet for supplies. The sound of the fetal heart monitor provides its steady *pock! pock! pock!*

"Okay, now," says Resident Karen Hill with warm enthusiasm. "Let's go ahead and check you at the end, okay?"

"Yeah," says Lily, her voice somewhat muffled by the oxygen mask's green plastic barrier. "Sure."

"Because I bet you it's time to really push," continues the resident. She sits on the edge of the operating table and plunges her right arm between Lily's massive thighs, deep within the patient's vagina.

"I hope I'm not hurting you, Lily," says the doctor from behind her mask.

Lily shakes her head: uh-uh.

"Yeah," says Karen Hill. "That cervix is gone! Now give me a big *push*, Lily! Big *push!*"

"*Uuuuungh!*" grunts the patient.

"That's the way—good!" responds the doctor. "Attaway! Good! Push-push-push-push-*push* that baby!"

"*Ooooooooh!*" moans the huge and laboring woman.

"*Push* that baby!" repeats the resident.

"Let's have another push," says the blond nurse, standing now alongside the operating table.

"C'mon, baby! You can do it!" Lily Pratt's husband, at last, speaks.

"*Ooooooooh!*" moans Lily. "*Uuuuungh!*"

"C'mon—you're doing it, you're doing it!" cheers the resident. "Wonderful! Wonderful!"

"*Uuuuungh!*"

The contraction is over, the *pock! pock! pock!* has slowed, and sweat is rolling off Lily's brow. David Pratt reaches into his pocket for an ironed, blazing-white handkerchief. Carefully, he wipes his wife's face.

Pock! pock! pock! The baby's heart rate is increasing, another contraction on its way.

"Another one! Can you go again?" asks Karen Hill.

Pock-pock-pock-pock-pock!

This baby wants out!

Lily pushes. And pushes. And pushes.

"Good! Good! Wonderful! Wonderful!" says the resident, laughing.

"Is it all right?" asks Lily.

"Oh, yeah," replies Karen Hill. "You're doing it! Wonderful! *Push* that baby! C'mon, *push* that baby! Good! Good!"

"Attaway, baby!" croons Lily's husband.

"*Ooooooooh!*" says his wife.

"Wonderful!" says Karen Hill. "Okay, c'mon! Give me another *push*! You've still got a contraction! Good! Good!"

"Attaway, baby!" chimes in David Pratt.

"*Uuuuungh!*" says Lily. It is a sound somewhere between a moan of agony and a scream. "I'm sorry!" She is mortified by the noises she realizes are coming from herself.

"Now, now," soothes the resident. "*All* women do that, okay?"

"I'm sorry!" repeats the patient, beginning to cry. "I'm sorry!" Soft sobs through the oxygen mask fill the room.

Pock! pock! pock! pock! pock! filters the baby's heartbeat through the monitor.

"It's okay," says David Pratt to his wife.

"Having a baby isn't exactly a polite experience, Lily," says Resident Karen Hill. "Okay?"

"Yeah," says the patient.

"Want to give me a little more push?" asks the doctor.

"What do you want me to do now?" is the plaintive answer.

"Just rest now, because your contraction is over, actually," says Karen Hill.

It isn't.

Pock-pock-pock-pock-pock!

"Oooooh! Oooooh! Oooooh!"

"I still think it's coming," says Nurse Becky Abramson. "It might last."

"Here I go again," announces Lily.

"Got a contraction?" asks the doctor.

"*Oooooh,* yes!"

"C'mon! *Push* that baby! *Push* that baby! *Push* that baby! *PUSH*!" chants Dr. Hill.

"*Oooooh!*"

"Push with the contraction," urges the nurse. "*Push!*"

"*Oooooh!*" moans Lily Pratt. Now, a full octave higher: "*Oooooh! Oooooh! Oooooh!*" She screams. A primal grunt follows, a bellow, a sound like her body is trying to expel an object too large for its exit point. (Which, as any woman who's been through labor knows, it is.)

"Make it a long, steady pushing," instructs the nurse. "That's right."

"Can I use a stirrup or something?" asks the patient.

"Yeah, we can do that," replies Dr. Hill. She turns to the nurse: "I don't want her flat on her back. I'll just put one shoulder against her leg."

"If I can just have one leg up..." pleads Lily.

"Yeah, I'm going to get one up," says Dr. Hill.

"...'cause, see, I need something to push down with."

"Yeah, we'll see if we can get some support here for your leg," continues her doctor.

Lily Pratt sighs, rearranging her body on the operating table in OR2. She pants heavily.

"Am I doing good?" she asks.

"Yes," says Dr. Karen Hill. "You're doing *wonderful!*"

Pock-pock-pock-pock-pock! With the approaching contraction, the baby's heartbeat speeds up. Lily waves away the doctor and nurse who are rearranging the position of her right leg.

"I don't have time for that," she tells them. "Here comes one!"

"Okay," says the nurse, "give us a push!"

"*Uuuuungh!*" she grunts. "Give me something to hang *on* to!"

"Give us a *push*," repeats the nurse.

"Push-push-push-push-push-push-push!" Dr. Hill cheers her on. "Push *hard*! C'mon, push *hard*! Oh, you're doing *great*!"

"*Uuuuungh!*" Lily replies. "*Oooooh! Uuuuungh!*"

"*Push* that baby! *Push* that baby! *Push* that baby! *All RIGHT!*" says Karen Hill.

Lily Pratt screams.

"*Push* that baby! *Push* that baby! *Push* that baby! *All RIGHT!*"

Again, Lily screams.

Dr. Hill turns to the nurse and murmurs a request for something from the supply cabinet.

Lily, her contraction over, sighs heavily.

"Okay," says Dr. Hill, "just rest. Just rest. Your baby is *very* close here. *Very* close."

"Is it crowning?" Lily asks.

"Not quite," Karen Hill answers. "But it's not going to be long. You're bringing him down *real nice* here."

The resident and the nurse consult quietly. The baby's

heart tones are down, and the next few minutes will determine whether they have to section Lily. Dr. Karen Hill speaks to the patient:

"With the next contraction, I want you to really push it down."

"Here it comes!" Lily announces.

"Okay! Give 'er a *push*! Give 'er a *push*! You can *do* it! You can *do* it!" Dr. Hill is back into cheerleader mode.

Everyone talks together, urging Lily on.

David Pratt: "Here goes! *Push,* honey, *push*! Push it *w-a-a-a-a-y* out!"

Dr. Karen Hill: "C'mon! *You* can do it! *You* can do it!"

Nurse Becky Abramson: *"Push-push-push-push-PUSH!"*

Lily: *"Oooooh! Uuuuungh! Oooooh, it hurts!"*

"That's right, Lily," agrees Dr. Hill. "It's going to hurt a little bit!"

"Oooooh! Uuuuungh!"

"It's okay—you can do it!" continues the resident.

"It's okay, honey. It's moving down now," David Pratt tells her.

Looking into her husband's face, Lily moans and shudders.

"Am I doing all right?" she asks. "Is it moving when I push?"

"Give me a push. A real long push. Deep and long," instructs the doctor. "C'mon, keep it coming! Keep it coming! *Push* that baby, *push* that baby, *push* that baby! *Push-push-push-push-push-PUSH!"*

"Eeeeeuuuuungh!"

"Hold your breath and *push*!" persists Dr. Hill. "Your breath is your power! Your breath is your power! Keep *pushing*!"

"Eeeeeuuuuungh!"

"Take a deep breath and *push,"* says the nurse. "Long and deep! Hold it down as long as you can!"

The contraction is over, and Dr. Hill tells Lily to rest. The doctor decides to use the Mityvac suction device.

"Your power," she tells Lily, "is in your breathing. If you hold your breath in and push, that gives you more power to push, okay?"

Behind the green oxygen mask, Lily nods in under-standing.

"Now I really need you to work hard at it because your baby's heart tone is not terribly low, but it's kind of tending to be low. We need to get this baby out kind of fast. Okay?"

Again, a nod from Lily.

"I'm going to use a little suction cup to put on the baby's head—to kind of help things along. So that when you push, I'll just give a little traction on this little suction cup on baby's head. Okay?"

Lily nods as she is borne off on the wave of a fresh contraction.

Pock-pock-pock-pock-pock!

"Uuuuungh! Uuuuungh!"

"Okay, here comes your next contraction," says David Pratt, unnecessarily.

"If it's coming, *push!*" says Karen Hill. "Push for all you're worth, Lily! OK? Push for all you're worth!"

"Uuuuungh! Uuuuungh!"

The clock on the wall behind the table in OR2 says it's 4:31 P.M.

Pock-pock-pock-pock-pock!

"Uuuuungh! Uuuuungh! Uuuuungh!"

"Longer, longer," says Nurse Becky Abramson. "Not the little grunts. Push for as long as you can!"

"Uuuuungh-uuuuungh- UUUUUNGH!"

Pock-pock-pock-pock-pock!

Lily screams.

"Keep 'em coming, baby," yells David Pratt.

Lily screams again.

"Good! Good!" says Dr. Hill. "Push! Push! Okay, okay—help me out, Lily! Keep 'em coming! Give me a nice push! Give me a nice push!"

"Uuuuungh! Uuuuungh! Uuuuungh!"

Lily Pratt, in her pink plissé nightie with the rosebuds, is among people whom (with the exception of her husband) she will never see again after this foggy April afternoon. Yet, lying here on a cold table in a public hospital on top of a hill in the agonizing throes of advanced labor, Lily has never felt more safe, more surrounded by love, in all her life. Finally, finally, she is *like other people*.

Embarrassment gone, Lily yawps and roars and screeches her harsh song of childbirth, as her mother did in birthing her eight children long ago, and *as her* mother did before her.

Dr. Karen Hill: "*Push! Push! Push! Push!*"

Nurse Becky Abramson: "*Push! Push! Push! Push!*"

David Pratt: "*Atta girl!*"

"She didn't have an epidural, did she?" the doctor asks the nurse.

She didn't.

Time for an episiotomy.

"Could we have some Betadine here?" the resident asks the nurse. Soaking a gauze sponge with the lurid orange disinfecting solution, Dr. Hill cleans Lily's vaginal area, downward toward the anus.

"Am I doing good?" Lily asks.

"Yep, yep, yep!" says the doctor. "Now, you're going to feel a little pick here. Just a little pick."

She injects the numbing lidocaine.

"*Oh! Oh! Oh! Oh!*" says Lily. "I felt that!"

After waiting for the drug to take effect, Dr. Hill uses the special episiotomy scissors to slice through the perineum, creating an exit door large enough for the baby to emerge. Lily begins to quake, making short little moans.

"Are you having another contraction now?" asks the resident.

"No," replies the patient, then swiftly changes her mind. "Oh, yes, I am!"

"Give me another *push*," she is instructed. "Give me a *push*! C'mon—hard as you can! Hard as you can! C'mon!"

"*Long and hard! Long and hard! Long and hard!*" (This, from Becky, the nurse.)

"G-o-o-o-o-o, *baby*!" says David.

"*Uuuuungh! Uuuuungh! Uuuu-uuu-UUUNGH!*"

"*Good job!*" says Karen Hill. "And *again*! Just like that one! *Just like that one!*"

"*Uuuuungh! Uuuuungh! Uuuu-uuu-UUUNGH!*"

"Push-push-push-push-push-PUSH that baby!"

Lily screams. She grunts. She moans.

"Oh, *God*! Oh, *God*! Oh, *God*!"

"*Keep it coming! Keep it coming! Keep it coming!*" says Resident Karen Hill.

"*Here it comes! Here it comes! Here it comes!*" says Nurse Becky Abramson.

Lily Pratt moans. Somewhere deep in her swirling mind, she thinks: *How can I do this?* Her body is flying apart, shredding into slivers, exploding into smithereens. What her mouth says is this:

"*Eeeeeungh! Oh, God! Ooooooh!*"

"Good! Good! Wonderful!" says her doctor.

"It's here, it's here!" says her nurse.

"Oh, baby, baby, baby!" says her husband, who has dropped Lily's hand to see his son's head push its way into the world.

"It's all right, Lily," says Dr. Karen Hill. "He's out now!"

"Very good!" says the blond nurse.

"A wonderful baby! A wonderful little boy!" says Karen Hill.

"Oh, Jesus!" says the new father. "There's our little boy!"

"Oh!" says Lily, oxygen mask gone from her face, laughing as tears course down her full cheeks. "Oh! Oh! Oh!"

The newborn inhales deeply and begins screaming. Everyone laughs, and the child is handed over to the pediatrics team at the side of OR2.

Someone opens the door from the nurses' station in the hall outside and asks: "Well?"

"Baby's out," confirms Karen Hill. "Boy at 1634." Peds has finished their initial examination of the newborn, and a nurse carries him to the head of the table in OR2 and shows him to Lily.

"Ooooooh!" says Lily, with a great shuddering cry. "Oh, *dearest*!" She laughs and laughs and laughs, her large body quaking with primal pleasure.

"At 4:34, you became a mom," says her weeping husband, kissing her in solemn formality: first the damp left cheek, then the right one.

"And at 4:34, you became a dad," replies his wife, stroking his cheek with her right index finger, repeating the tender gesture then on both cheeks of their son. "Oh, sweetie!" She cries and cries and laughs and laughs as the infant continues to scream.

"Baby looking great!" announces Dr. Karen Hill, whose eyes are red-rimmed.

"Oh thank you, Lord," says the new mother, looking heavenward.

"Congratulations," says Nurse Becky Abramson.

"Thank you for everything," says Lily, looking from the doctor to the nurse and back again, smiling smiling smiling. The nurse gently removes the baby to continue the newborn's routine.

Scott David Pratt continues to cry.

He weighs six pounds and three ounces. Not the ten or eleven pounds everyone thought!

"Don't he sound *cute*, David?" Lily asks her husband.

Now, Dr. Hill tells her patient, they have to wait for the placenta to deliver, then there'll be "a little bitty episiotomy thing to sew up."

"Fine," says Lily. Everything is fine now. Everything everything fine fine fine.

"Congratulations, Lily," the doctor continues. "You did a wonderful job there with your pushing. Got that baby out so fast I couldn't believe it!"

"Oh, he sounds so sweet! Is he okay?" Lily asks.

"He's just fine," Second-Year Resident Karen Hill assures her. "He's a wonderful baby."

CHAPTER ELEVEN

("I believe there is some discomfort associated with pregnancy," says the chief resident.)

1705: 5:05 P.M.

DARLEEN ROBINSON, REFERRED TO up on 4NE as "last night's seizure disorder," lies in her bed in the Mother-Baby Unit, recovering from the emergency c-section that brought forth a 7½-pound boy at nine this morning. After long hours of labor (with her stern mother continuing her imperturbable rocking and reading of religious tracts), Darleen's fetal heart monitor strip showed deep decelerations of the baby's heart rate, and the decision was made to perform a cesarean.

"It's hard work, but when you think about it, that's what we wanted, wasn't it, honey?" Darleen asks her husband, who has just returned from going home to shower and change.

"Yeah, I guess so," he replies, regarding without expression his son in the bassinet.

In the room next door to Darleen Robinson, Alison Gill contemplates her future as she nurses her 8½-pound daughter. Sure, she could stay in Portland with her mom and Tom and her idiot twin sister. But Darryl has called her three times already today, and says he'll drive here from Reno next weekend. She only wishes she knew him better. A funny thing to say about the father of your child!

It was last summer that Alison and her sister Charlene (monkeys will fly out her butt before *she* calls her Jasmine, for crying out loud!) went to visit their grandmother in Reno for a month. Well, one day when Charlene was doing her nails and didn't want to go on a walk with her, Alison met Darryl, who lives just down the street from her grandmother, and they started going out together, and one night after they went to see a movie, they were making out in the back of Darryl's old Toyota Corolla station wagon that he got for $500, and one thing just led to another, you know? When Alison went home in August, Darryl promised to write, but he never did.

When she had missed two periods, Alison finally talked to her mom, who was real nice about it, and she even told Alison she didn't want her to have an abortion or give up the baby for adoption, either. "This is my grandbaby, Alison," she kept saying. "In this family, we take care of our own!" Her stepfather was upset for about an hour after she told him. "I'm gonna kill that little sonofabitch!" he shouted, walking back and forth in the living room, with the Channel 8 news just going on and on, but nobody paying any attention to it. But then Alison's stepdad was real sweet about it. ("Are you *okay*, honey?" he kept asking. "Are you *okay*?") And her mom, she was great. She sat Alison down and helped her write a letter to Darryl.

Was Alison ever surprised when Darryl just plain showed up at the door only three days after she mailed that letter to Reno! He stayed with her family for two whole days, all the time trying to talk her into getting married (and her still in high school!). Her family really liked him except Charlene, who stayed in her room and acted like she was mad most of the time he was here.

The plan they worked out was that Darryl would go back to school in Reno, where he's a sophomore in pre-law, and that after the baby came, if she wanted to, Alison would move to Reno to live with him and his parents. His mom called Alison, and she sounded real nice. Then she talked to Alison's mom and told her something Darryl doesn't know (and made her *promise* not to tell him), that he was born only five months after she and his dad got married!

Alison doesn't know what to do. I mean, how do you even know you're in love, you know?

"What do you think we ought to do, Amanda Jayne?" Alison asks her baby. "Shall we go live with your daddy?"

The newborn, who Alison thinks looks so much like Darryl that it's a little bit creepy, just keeps on nursing.

1750: 5:50 P.M.

It's raining now, drizzling like it was January instead of mid-April. A medical student sits at the table in the coffee/supply room, reading the funnies as she grabs another oatmeal cookie (spices! raisins! big chunks of walnuts!) from a polka-dotted red metal tin with a picture of a quilt on the lid. Nurses Susan Cech and Becky Abramson are drinking strong coffee of a certain age, saying how glad they are that Lily Pratt went vaginally. And they talk about how the other residents are going to give Nicky-Nicky Abrudescu a hard time for bailing out on Lily, once he gets back from vacation.

Vicky Cohen, a nurse-midwife from one of the county satellite clinics, is talking with Dr. Richard Lowensohn out in the hallway. Tonight, Dr. Kirk is staffing. But in the weekend ahead, on both Saturday and Sunday, it will be Dr. Lowensohn's turn to oversee the residents on duty on 4NE.

At forty-four, Dr. Lowensohn looks like someone in charge. He is short of stature, small in build, his bearing dignified, almost military. The dark moustache is neatly trimmed, bald head as polished as the black shoes below his green scrubs. His official title is Chief of Obstetrics, Director of the Division of Maternal Fetal Medicine, and Associate Professor of Obstetrics and Gynecology. Like all the other faculty members in Pill Hill's OB/GYN Department, he takes his turn on L&D, keeping his eye on the residents, monitoring the decisions made by the chiefs, interfering as little as possible.

Dick Lowensohn grew up in Los Angeles, the son of an OB/GYN, and was constantly asked: "So, you're going to be a doctor like your father, right?" His answer, always, was,

159

"Wrong!" Instead, he thought he'd be an engineer, like his grandfather. He had decided to compromise, to go into medical electronics, when, halfway through his engineering education, he was struck by the realization that it was just as silly *not* to be a doctor because your father is one, as it is to *be* a doctor because your father is one. So, he added pre-med courses to his curriculum while continuing with the engineering training.

He went to med school, and did his residency at University of Southern California. After doing a fellowship in maternal fetal medicine, Dr. Lowensohn stayed on the USC faculty for a year, taught at the University of Chicago for five years, tried a private practice in perinatology in Berkeley for three years.

But he found he missed the research, missed the teaching, missed being around the residents. A few years earlier, he'd almost come to OHSU, to be a team leader with Dr. Kirk in his pre-chairman years. He called Pill Hill and asked if there was an opening. His timing was good, and he was hired. That was a year and a half ago.

There's a lot of public health care here, and that's a big part of what Dr. Lowensohn likes about his job. He can try to come up with prevention programs, with interventions, with better ways to handle certain things. For example, after a review of how to deal with patients with a history of herpes, they ended up stopping doing a culture every week from thirty-four weeks on. It costs a lot of money per patient to do those weekly cultures, and it turned out they didn't help, anyway. Once he found that out, he was eager to put that money to better use.

There are frustrations, God knows. The tap-dancing-on-the-edge feeling, the constant surges of adrenaline, are exciting. But you pay too heavily when it's over, and your family pays, too. One of the reasons Dick Lowensohn came up to Oregon was to have a better life with his family. He has two young children, five and nine years old. He doesn't intend to get swallowed up in this, to the point where the better life doesn't happen.

Here's where it's happening. If he changes the way residents approach patients, then he's changing the way thousands of patients get taken care of in the coming years.

With public health obstetrics, a lot of the problem is getting women to show up for prenatal care on time, to really get involved with their own pregnancies. What Dr. Lowensohn wants to do is to organize some sort of consumer-directed campaign. Like basic propaganda with attractive rebates or whatever it takes to make pregnant women come in for their appointments. A lot of those no-shows might show up because they get some personal reward for doing it. They might respond to something at that level.

There are so many problems. Take the sheer patient volume overload. Doctors in private practice pay incredibly high malpractice premiums, and they don't want to take on a lot of new patients who are going to spell trouble. Just by screening for insurance, their office help shields them from ever having to say, "Don't come here." So a lot of women don't get prenatal care, not because someone is literally sending them away, but because they're not allowed through the door in the first place. So they just show up here, take a bus, hitch a ride, trudge somehow up that hill when they get in trouble. They show up whether they're in trouble or not, just show up in labor.

The med school's charter from the state doesn't say anything about providing indigent care. So there is no state money in the department budget that specifically covers indigent care. For that matter, there's no money coming from anyplace else for indigent care, either.

Yet Pill Hill functions as the state hospital that does indigent care. If you're the county hospital, then a chunk of what you do is care for indigent patients. What the state does provide is a fairly small amount of money earmarked for teaching. In order to teach residents, you have to bring in a certain number of patients with X condition for doctors and nurses to get experience in dealing with that condition. Not all of those patients are going to have money or insurance. So the state allows a certain number of dollars to care for those X-condition patients, but it's really, officially anyway, to provide the residents with the training they need.

That's all very well and good. Except, of course, that there's nowhere near enough money to slip every indigent patient in under the wire. The state funds have to be spread

161

around over all the departments. This many patients aren't essential for simple teaching purposes. Yet you can't turn them away: No one else will take them. And one of the reasons Pill Hill can "afford" them is because its malpractice insurance is covered by the state.

There are not enough people to take care of all the women who come here to have their babies. Dr. Lowensohn doesn't want to expand the residency to be large enough to handle the obstetrical load. There needs to be some resolution that doesn't overload the residents any more than they already are. As it is, the overload means the residents aren't being taught as much as they could be, because they don't have the time to come to the teaching sessions. Sure, they're getting plenty of hands-on experience, but not enough teaching. Dr. Lowensohn can come up with the time to teach them. So can the rest of the faculty. It's the residents who can't come up with the time.

The hospital administration would like the OB/GYN Department to change the patient mix, to bring in a lot more private patients. Paying patients. But with the shape 4NE is in, how can they? Especially when the comparison is with Good Samaritan, or St. Vincent's, with their champagne dinners and their plush carpeting and their no-drug-addicts-in-the-room next-door. Pill Hill will never be able to get rid of the drug addicts in the room next door. If some things can get changed, some people might be willing to come here. Just because it is the university. Just because it might be a little safer. But compete with those other hospitals? Fat chance.

The way Dr. Lowensohn looks at it, the private hospitals owe OHSU in a big way. Pill Hill is helping the private hospitals stay competitive with one another. It's *because* of the heavy load of indigent patients up on Pill Hill that Good Sam and St. Vincent's and the others have pretty halls, uncluttered with low-income families and their undesirable families. Go have your baby at Good Samaritan, and you're almost guaranteed not to room next door to a drug addict.

Because the private doctors never see indigent cases (and let's face it, the reason patients end up at private hospitals is because of their private doctors), Portland's other hospitals don't do their share of indigent care. Those private hospitals owe OHSU something. A tax based on their proportional share of the number of indigent patients they're *not* taking care of. Fair's fair.

1810: 6:10 P.M.

Fili, the hospital aide, mops the floor out by the nurses' station as staff Dr. Mark Nichols is on the phone, telling his wife he can't, as promised, take their small son to the movies tonight, after all. Kathy Dahlstrom, his private patient, has been pushing for four hours, and her baby is still too high up. So they're going to have to section her, and Dr. Nichols will be supervising the residents performing the surgery.

Two medical students talk about Darleen Robinson, the "seizure disorder" crash-sectioned this morning. She's down on the third floor, in "Muh-Boo," the Mother-Baby Unit.

"I was down in Muh-boo this afternoon, and the baby was crying, and she said, 'Shut up, or I'll slap you!'" says one student to the other.

"I heard it, too," says Nurse Susan Cech, overhearing the students. "Maybe the CSD should be alerted, and should make a home visit?" Arrangements are made to contact the Children's Services Division, the state's child protection agency.

1827: 6:27 P.M.

Kathy Dahlstrom, Dr. Nichols's private patient, is a nurse. She's familiar with most of the procedures preparing her for her cesarean section: the epidural anesthesia, the pulling of the drape so that she can't see the surgery in progress, the gathering of doctors, nurses, and the handsome medical student who's acting as scrub technician. The surgery is done by Resident Karen Hill, who delivered Lily Pratt's baby a scant two hours ago.

163

A beautiful baby girl, not a mark on her, is scooped out of Kathy's belly.

1930: 7:30 P.M.

In Room 16, Carmen Ramirez is exhausted from her first labor. She's been in Labor and Delivery through all shifts today, and the belief is that the cord is wrapped around her baby's neck. Hot, exhausted breath steams up her transparent green oxygen mask as Nurse Jeanne Gates smiles and massages the patient's huge belly, chanting: "*Sopla! Sopla! Sopla!*"

Breathe! Breathe! Breathe!

In the small room outside the staff bathroom, beautiful little Annalise Dahlstrom, one hour old, is being weighed. She is flawless and beautiful, unusual for a person a mere hour outside the womb, and looks particularly fetching in her tiny pink knit cap. Receiving an injection, she waits several full seconds, looks amazed, then screws up her face and screams bloody murder.

2027: 8:27 P.M.

In Room 16, Medical Student Lorie Morgan, supervised by pregnant Resident Tracey Delaplain, delivers, at last, the Ramirez baby. Tracey, who has been awake and at the hospital since six yesterday morning, feels as though she is watching a movie. She's awake, all right, and alert. But everything seems brightly colored, sharp-edged.

"*Como se llama?*" asks Nurse Jeanne Gates. "What's his name?"

"*Se llama Jesús,*" replies the mother, weak but smiling. "*Jesús. Como su padre.*" Like his father.

As she is being taken down the hall to the INCU, little Jesús, covered from head to toe with a fine, dark down, is followed by beaming Jesús *grande.* While the nurses and peds resident do all the fussy bits, the shy father reaches out a tentative index finger to stroke his child.

"Eh?" he asks, nodding toward the baby. "Okay?"

"Sure," says a nurse. "You can touch him—he's yours!"

2048: 8:48 P.M.

Chief Resident Liz Newhall, for some reason wearing a white jacket with AUTOPSY PATHOLOGY stitched across the pocket in red, on her way over to X-Ray in South Hospital to check on an ultrasound, passes Nurse Susan Cech bringing a big bowl of microwaved popcorn toward the coffee/supply room.

Halfway to X-Ray, Liz's beeper goes off to check back with L&D. Grabbing the nearest phone, she's told there's a crash section in the offing for Karla Michaels. Like a bat out of hell, she runs back to 4NW.

Everyone is rushing into OR2 as the message goes out over the phone: "Dr. Kirk! Please call Labor and Delivery! We have a potential crash section! Dr. Kirk, please call Labor and Delivery...."

In the operating room, Karla Michaels is on her hands and knees on the operating table, a position that it is hoped will take the weight off the aorta and vena cava. Also, if the fetal distress is due to a compressed or prolapsed umbilical cord, this position will take the weight off the cervix and lower uterine section.

2110: 9:10 P.M.

In Room 8, the petulant Joni Phillips has a fever, and Chief Resident Liz Newhall is afraid the baby, whose tracings show a heart rate of 200, may be sick. Earlier, in the afternoon, it was thought that the accelerations were a result of Joni's asthma medication. Now, Liz isn't so sure.

"There must be something wrong," says Joni. "I feel shitty!"

"I believe there is some discomfort associated with pregnancy," calmly replies the chief resident.

"And I want my tubes tied!" says Joni.

"Honey!" This bleak cry comes from her husband, a small, plump man of perhaps thirty, and not the father of her first two children.

"I *do*, Cal! Don't give me any more *shit* about this!"

With a huge sigh, Cal leans back in his chair, evidently not planning to give his wife any more shit about this. At least not while that tall, redheaded doctor is in the room.

2135: 9:35 P.M.

In OR2 a scalp pH on Karla Michaels's baby shows the fetus to be okay, after all. The decision is made to let nature take its course. She is now getting an epidural.

Out in the hall, by the nurses' station, a sweet-faced and stout middle-aged woman, clad in tight shiny black double-knit pants and a swirly flower-printed overblouse, grips a bunch of tired daisies with her plump fingers and asks after Karla.

"When can I see her?" asks the woman. "She's my daughter!"

In the Exam Room, Sandi Scott, halfway along with her third child, is worried. Every fifteen minutes or so she's been getting this weird pain, she tells Liz Newhall. In her second pregnancy, she had a torsed ovary—a twist compromising the blood supply—with a cyst on it. Dr. Newhall leaves the room and returns a moment later, deftly hauling the ultrasound machine through the door after her.

The largish machine features a screen that looks like a computer monitor or a small TV screen. Sandi Scott's sleeveless pastel gingham plaid smock is pulled up, the elastic waistband of her hot-pink pedal pushers pulled in the opposite direction to reveal her high, round abdomen. Dr. Newhall squeezes out a long worm of pale green gel onto the surface of the patient's belly.

"Oooooh! Weird—and *cold*!" says Sandi Scott, laughing nervously.

"Yeah. Well, it helps the sound waves go through," says

the chief resident. She takes the ultrasound machine's transducer, which looks like a vacuum cleaner attachment at the end of a thick cord extending from the machine, and smears the gel across the pregnant woman's belly. The transducer sends a brief pulse of sound—about a millionth of a second long—into Sandi Scott's body. The pulse travels into her abdomen, reaches the outer surface of the uterus, and bounces back a little echo. Reaching the baby within, it sends another echo, and an image appears on the machine's TV monitor.

On the screen, the image is open to interpretation. If, say, you are one of those people who usually recognize the face of the man in the moon, if you see lambs and dragons in a skyful of white clouds, you could easily make out the shape of a very young human growing cozily in his mother's womb.

"See?" asks Liz Newhall. "There? Where the X is? That's his nose! And see there?" She moves the X a little distance, to the right. "He's sucking his thumb!"

"You're kidding!" says Sandi Scott.

"Well, I'll be!" says her husband.

Everything looks okay. Just fine.

"Oooooh! Is that really his *hand*?" Sandi Scott stares, entranced by the picture of her son on the screen, and with tears in her eyes.

"As long as we're doing the *ooooh! ah!* tour, you want a picture?" asks the chief resident.

"Oh, *could* I?" asks Sandi Scott.

"Sure—why not?" Liz Newhall prints out an ultrasound picture of Sandi Scott's hardy little *in utero* swimmer, his thumb firmly planted in his mouth.

2238: 10:38 P.M.

In the nursery, Jesús Ramirez works his arms and legs around, making peculiar little grunting noises, while in the INCU's other room, Timothy Edwards, born Monday in the ambulance, stiffens as a nurse picks him up to attempt to feed him. The infant has made progress this week. Now, at least, he will suck on the nipple. The Children's Services Division,

167

alerted earlier in the week, has set in motion a request for immediate termination of Cammie Edwards's parental rights, and is making plans for foster care for the tiny drug addict.

2244: 10:44 P.M.

In Room 8, Joni Phillips, chilling out her husband, zaps the TV set until she finds Pink Panther cartoons on Channel 49. Her husband stands at the window, glumfaced, looking out at the parking lot in the gray rain.

In Room 10, on Channel 2 Barbara Walters makes someone cry on the screen as Dr. Liz Newhall tells a spectacled young woman with a spiky black punk haircut that she can go home if she promises to come back if there's any bleeding or abdominal discomfort.

First-Year Resident Linda Moore, twenty-seven, tall and slim, pretty and black, stands at the nurses' station, glancing over the chart of Room 2's Clarice Morgan, just up from the Mother-Baby Unit. The baby is breech, the labor not well along, and the patient is loudly insisting she needs a cesarean section, and she needs it now. Tonight.

Like everyone else, the intern is tired, jacked up on coffee and sugar. But (like the others, too) she is glad, very glad, to be where she is. She has a nice apartment in West Slope, and every so often she gets to go skiing, either downhill or cross-country. Not that there's much social life to speak of. And what there is, is at the expense of sleep. Seems like every time she gets comfortable, makes some friends, maybe finds a romantic possibility, it's time to pack her bags and leave again.

Linda Moore was raised in Hawaii, the second of four kids of a general contractor and his wife, a nurse. She always did well in school. For a while, she thought about becoming a veterinarian, but became discouraged when she realized how badly people treat their animals, bringing them in only when they're really, really sick. (Funny, though. When she got into "real medicine," Linda discovered that's exactly what people do with their own bodies, too!)

Growing up in Hawaii, with its rainbow of different races,

Linda Moore didn't even know what racial prejudice was. Certainly, she never felt it. And when she came to the mainland to go to college, she spent a wonderful four years at Stanford University. Then came med school at the University of California at San Diego. There she got it, full force, pow-right-in-the-kisser.

A first-year medical school professor decided Linda shouldn't be in medicine, and did everything he could to flush her out. At first, she was hurt, perplexed. She was a nice person. She had never hurt anyone, never done anything to this man. Asking around, she found it was his practice to pick on the black and Hispanic students. Even though her cumulative score was higher than half of the rest of that first-year class, the professor made her repeat the year.

Linda petitioned up the wazoo, to no avail. What else could she do? That second year, she took second-year courses, while repeating the first year, which gave her a crushing course load. And she did very well, worked her butt off. Who knows what would have happened if she hadn't had the support of her family and friends, who kept giving her reality doses, assuring her she was right and he was wrong? The professor had money, big research bucks, and a big name. To him, the students were just transients passing through—and he was going to be there forever. When he found out she had doubled up, he was upset. Harassed her the whole time, told her if she didn't pass his course, she would be kicked out of med school. When he found out she was succeeding, he went to the microbiology department chair and told him he shouldn't let her take the exams together—because what if she passed? The microbiology guy told him off.

It was miserable. With the double course load, she'd sometimes have two or three exams the same week. In the middle of the night, she'd be so tired, wondering why she was torturing herself. Her friends would tell her why: because the prof was wrong and you don't want him to say, "I told you so." That strengthened her, gave her the perverse, angry energy she needed to pick up the books and study some more. Linda Moore passed all her courses, all of them. With flying colors.

When it came time for residency interviews, what could

she say about the first-year course she supposedly "failed"? She couldn't talk about racial discrimination, couldn't have them think, "Oh, God, one of *those,* saying that all her life's problems are because of her race!" Nope. She didn't bring up the racial crap. Instead, she just said there'd been some problems, and she had to redo the course, and did okay. Period.

Asshole.

Walking into Room 2, First-Year Resident Linda Moore is cool, professional, detached. She gives Clarice Morgan, up from MBU, a vaginal exam. Med Student Cynthia Fairfax paces at the foot of the bed as Clarice, wincing and starting with the pain, tells Dr. Moore that she's worried about the baby being breech.

"You're not having a real functional contraction pattern," Linda Moore tells the hard-faced couple. "And for that reason, we'd like to stop the labor. But we don't do things *to* you—it's a joint effort."

The hospital, she explains, is in a real bind for space, and Clarice would just have to be sent to another hospital.

"I want a c-section, so I can have my tubes tied at the same time," says the patient. Clearly, she hasn't heard a word said to her in the past few minutes.

"Well, with a vaginal birth, you can just have your tubes tied the next day," explains the resident.

The patient is adamant.

"Him and I," she says, gesturing her head toward her husband, "we both agree. There just is something wrong with having a *breech* baby vaginally!" She nods her head for emphasis: *so there!*

"Well, I'm a breech baby, and I was born vaginally, and *I'm* perfectly all right," says the black resident.

Patient and husband, aghast, look at each other.

Who the hell does she think she is?

170

CHAPTER TWELVE

DAY 6: Saturday, April 16

("I'm scared to deliver this baby," says the nurse-midwife.)

1746: 5:46 P.M.

IT'S SATURDAY AFTERNOON, AND fine mist surrounds the buildings atop Pill Hill. Outside North Hospital, in the parking lot, the hot-pink rhododendrons are in full, lush bloom. As Nurse-Midwife Nancy Sullivan walks across the skyway on her way back from South Hospital's third-floor cafeteria, she doesn't notice the profuse blossoms on the cherry trees below. Through the mist, she can barely make out the river. Not a sign of either Mount Hood or Mount St. Helens.

This is supposed to be Nancy Sullivan's day off, but here she is in her lime-green scrubs, the too-big pants tied around her midsection like a sack of potatoes. A slight woman, her graying-brown hair cropped into a short shag, peering through big round-rimmed glasses, Nancy has come in to look after Julie O'Brien.

Nancy Sullivan was born to be a midwife. For a while, in fact for most of her growing-up years in West Virginia in the 1950s, Nancy—Hillenbrand she was then—thought she wanted to be a doctor. But good grades and all, she was dis-

171

couraged early on. At the University of Pennsylvania, she majored in English. Women were not exactly sought out by medical schools in those days. After all, they'd "only marry and have kids," and all that education would go down the drain: Every dollar spent educating a woman is one less dollar you have to throw down the drain. When her husband, Neal, was attending law school at the University of Texas, she was told by the med school there that there was little point in her applying. Even if she were accepted, she would need much better grades than the male students got, just to be kept on. When Neal finished law school, the couple decided to join the Peace Corps. They both taught English in Morocco—until Nancy became pregnant with twins. The Corps booted them out, shipping them straight back to the States.

Nancy's experience bearing twin daughters was dismal. Ordered to bed for the second half of her pregnancy, she finally gave birth, heavily drugged, in a cold, brightly lighted operating room, where her participation (except as the vessel containing the babies) seemed unnecessary, her very presence oddly extraneous.

It was only when the Sullivans were living in Paris, having been transferred there by the international oil company Neal worked for at the time, that Nancy realized what a natural, joyous event giving birth could be. In accordance with prevailing French medical custom, she was tended throughout her second pregnancy by a midwife—or *sage femme,* "wise woman." What a contrast with her experience with the twins in the Texas hospital! It was personal and loving, taking into account what Nancy and Neal wanted. Just as she began looking into midwifery training in Paris, Neal was transferred back to America, to New York City. Against the advice of everyone they knew, the Sullivans bought an apartment in Manhattan. (This was 1974, the year of the *New York Post* headline: FORD TO CITY: DROP DEAD!)

Knowing at last what she really wanted to do, Nancy began training to be a nurse-midwife, American style. She enrolled in Cornell University's nursing program, right around the corner from their new home, plunking small Patrick in the hospital's preschool. Two years later, nursing degree in hand, she worked at Roosevelt Hospital with the nurse-midwives

172

there, hoping to get approval for admission to Columbia University's prestigious nurse-midwifery program. Two years later, she was admitted to training.

In 1980 Nancy Sullivan finally became a midwife.

When the Sullivans decided that living in Manhattan was too dirty and too dangerous, and that the suburbs had no appeal, Neal got a job in Portland, working with an international maritime corporation. After a few months, Nancy began doing fill-in vacation relief midwifery work on Pill Hill. Before long, she was a staff member. And never, not for a moment, did she wish she were Nancy Sullivan, M.D.

In Labor and Delivery, it's one of those nights. All eight delivery rooms are full except for the Exam Room. Six women in advanced labor have already been "diverted" to other Portland hospitals: one to Adventist, another to St. V's, and the rest to Good Sam.

Snoozing off her anesthetic in PAR is Lisa Kubicek, four feet nine, thirty years old, and herself a triplet, who has just had her second child by cesarean section.

The Board says that twenty-seven-year-old Crystal Mooney, laboring in Room 16, has had two abortions, two live births, and one living child. She is also an intravenous drug abuser—and HIV positive.

In Room 18, Maria Veiera, a migrant worker who's been getting her prenatal care at Salud, Salem's county health clinic, is in the early stages of labor.

Diana Dante, in Room 10, is a private patient of Dr. Desmond Johnson. Her unborn baby is already dead, for reasons unknown, and she lies on her side, knees brought up as far as her thirty-four-week pregnancy will allow. Long and thin, with short curly blond hair, Diana is propped up with three pillows, facing the television set above as she waits for her induced labor to gather speed. Tears trickle down her blank face as *Star Trek*'s Captain Kirk, immortal in rerun, blurts out his suspicion that the leader of an acting troupe is really Kudos the Executioner, presumed dead for decades.

Tucked into Room 8, Teresa Nuñoz is well into the late stage of labor with her ninth child, and is being coached in Spanish by Nurse Jeanne Gates: *"Sopla! Sopla! Empuje!"* Push!

173

Marilee Babcock—thin and jittery and needing a fix *now*—has been sent home to wait for two days before the staff will induce the birth of her anencephalic baby, an infant with no brain.

Julie O'Brien, Nurse-Midwife Nancy Sullivan's patient, is still downstairs in the Mother-Baby Unit, and most of her crying is over. She is nearly eight months along, and a week ago an ultrasound revealed that her baby is only the size of a twenty-four-week-old fetus, weighing perhaps one pound or so. A subsequent amniocentesis revealed severe chromosomal abnormalities. The fetus is what's called "triploid"—one of its chromosome sets is duplicated, triploid instead of diploid. With no chance for a normal outcome, the decision has been made to induce, and thus terminate, the pregnancy.

And so, early this morning, three *laminaria* sticks were inserted into Julie's cervix. Made of seaweed fashioned into the size and shape of a kitchen matchstick, the laminaria have been absorbing fluid, over the hours expanding to the size of slender tampons. They have thinned and softened the cervix, encouraging labor to begin, which will effectively abort the pregnancy, probably before the evening ends. It has been decided that no heroic measures will be taken to extend the baby's life—if indeed it survives the trip down the birth canal. There will be no respirator present, though they'll hydrate the infant. They'll keep it warm, and that's comforting to Julie. ("It." Nice thing to call a baby, huh?)

Nobody knows quite what to expect. A triploid fetus can manifest abnormalities in a number of ways. Ears can be weirdly aligned, say, maybe placed way down toward, or even *on,* the neck. One form of chromosome abnormality results in Down's syndrome. Sometimes a triploid fetus has no arms or legs. The genitalia are often what's termed "ambiguous." Perinatologist Dr. Young told Nancy Sullivan that the ultrasound of Julie's baby looked like there was a clubfoot. Everyone—doctors, nurses, and Nancy herself—is pretty nervous, hoping however to stay professional and cool. Hoping they won't be too surprised, at least not visibly horrified, by whatever propels out of Julie's vagina when the time comes.

Julie O'Brien has spent most of her life heading the committee to make everyone else comfortable and happy. A lovely, sweet-faced thirty-one-year-old, with hair the color of a mellowed copper penny, she is organized in a solid, emotional way. She makes careful preparations, believes in God's Perfect Plan, and has taken care of every detail to make this horrible experience as okay as possible for everyone. Her red-haired eight-year-old is all set to bring treats to his Cub Scout meeting this afternoon. Her blond mother is flying in from D.C. Her black boyfriend, Maurice, more distant with each day of this unplanned pregnancy, has promised to show up and be with her. And her girlfriends Annette and Lori are all ready to come to Pill Hill to hold her hand during the worst of it all.

Julie has always been adaptable and outgoing. She was even an American Field Service exchange student to Costa Rica when she was sixteen. And Julie takes some satisfaction from knowing that she can love people and say good-bye to them, knowing that it has been an enriching experience. No matter who, no matter what it is.

But when she walked into the hospital yesterday morning, Julie's whole attitude changed. Her confidence collapsed, deflated with the dispatch of a kid's day-old helium-filled balloon. But there was Nancy Sullivan, who had seen her through it all—including that godawful afternoon when Maurice didn't show up for the amniocentesis results. Nancy was the one who put the lamanaria in, even on her day off, and stuck around for a couple of hours, just to be there for her. Never making her feel, you know, like she was imposing or something. Even when she went home, Nancy told Julie she only lived ten minutes away, and she'd come back when things got under way. And Julie knew the nurse-midwife meant it, from the heart.

For the past couple of years, Julie has been in a wonderful relationship with Maurice. (It may come as a shock to some people, being that they're both Christians and it's such a bad witness being pregnant outside of marriage, but you try your hardest and sometimes you fail.) However, as soon as she discovered she was pregnant, Maurice began to pull away. He knew that the ultrasound showed there might be problems with the baby, and he knew the worst of what that could mean. But still—*still*—he was a half hour late for getting the amnio test results. He wasn't there, and it was all over.

In fact, Julie was already driving off The Hill, sobbing

175

like crazy, and here comes Maurice, just moseying up in his sports car, driving *real* slow. That's when she thought, "You may think you're involved, mister, but as far as I'm concerned, you are uninvolved from this point forward." And then that night, the very same night after she learned their baby was going to be some kind of freak, he says, you know, that he's got to get back to work and if you need anything give me a call. And when she calls him all the way till four in the morning, and he still isn't home, when she needs him the most, Julie got to thinking that maybe Lori and Annette were right, after all. That Maurice wasn't all that involved with her. That *she* was the one in an exclusive relationship.

Outside Room 8, Teresa Nuñoz's husband, Javier, is pacing. When the door opens, he can hear Teresa crying out: "*Ay-ay-ay-ay-ay!*" He assures the nurses and doctors that he has no wish to enter the room where his wife is bringing forth their first child. Men do not belong with birthing women. Like his father and his grandfather and all other men in his family, all the men he knows, he will wait outside. But Teresa is so tiny and he worries. When the short, stocky farmworker is certain nobody can see him, Javier Nuñoz gnaws at what is left of his fingernails.

1812: 6:12 P.M.

Brought upstairs from the Mother-Baby Unit, lying now in her bed in L&D's Special Delivery Room, the largest and best of the six birthing rooms, Julie O'Brien is calm. She's been taking a lot of long, deep breaths. Her faith in the Lord Jesus Christ helps. All this is just part of God's Plan for her life. Right now, God has been gracious enough to give her the right amount of friends at the right time, and this is no time for moaning and complaining.

In the room, in addition to Julie are Annette and Lori, two of the best friends the Lord could have given anybody. Wonderful Annette, with her dark brown shag cut and open, trusting face. And blond, freckled Lori, who used to work with Julie as a checkout girl in a local supermarket, and who has two kids herself by a black man. With Nurse-Midwife Nancy Sullivan and Nurse Carolyn Bachhuber, they all listen to the frail baby's heartbeat, a gentle yet constant sound broadcast on the fetal heart monitor. The radio is tuned to KMHD, playing jazz from Mount Hood Community College's student-run station.

In the hall outside the room, Carolyn Bachhuber turns to Nancy Sullivan as the two make their way toward the coffee/supply room. Nancy tells Carolyn about Maurice's no-show for the amnio results.

"The bastard," she says.

"Men are *jerks*, you know that?" Carolyn asks the nurse-midwife.

1834: 6:34 P.M.

In the coffee/supply room, people are enjoying a brief quiet time. Talking about Crystal Mooney, laboring away in Room 16. Her baby will almost certainly be born drug-addicted, they agree. These things are predictable. You can tell. All you need to know is the first name of the mother. "Crystal" almost always. Same for "Angel" and "Tiffany." "Tammy" can go either way, though. With the young black mothers, it's harder to tell, since so many have the new made-up names. LaDawna. Tawneeta. Shereesha.

In Room 10, Resident Kathleen Doyle is telling Diana Dante that she might want something to ease the pain of her labor. Anything she will receive, Diana is told, will take thirty minutes to take hold. Back at the nurses' station, OB-GYN Dr. Desmond Johnson, Diana Dante's physician, jokes to a group of nurses.

"Laminaria," he says, "goes in small and comes out big . . . unlike anything else!" The women groan.

"*That*," says a nurse once he's out of earshot, "is why he no longer works here!"

Down in the Mother-Baby Unit, Lily Pratt, one large and happy woman, is explaining to three of her sisters about trying to nurse her new little son Scott. Lying in her bed, Lily laughs happily, frequently. All her sisters, like Lily, are large women, none under 300 pounds. They clamor for a chance to hold the sleeping child, but the new mother isn't ready to relinquish him just yet.

"You'll all have your turn soon enough," she says. "Just be patient!" Scott Pratt's father, David, sits beside the bed, watching and smiling, his head gently bobbing to an inner music only he can hear.

Upstairs in L&D, Julie O'Brien's labor is tuning up, starting to be real work. The patient is talking with her friend Annette about her son Josh. It's been a tough six months for him. Julie's ex-husband was always one of those I'm-in-love-with-my-kid-more-than-anything-in-the-world dads. Then, all of a sudden he remarries out of the blue and moves to Salt Lake City. Without any notice, without telling Josh, without even leaving a forwarding address. Then, she has to get rid of the cat because Josh starts having all these allergy problems. Then, the new canary she gets him dies after a month. And now this, his little sister or brother he was looking forward to so much.

Julie turns to the nurse-midwife. She wants to know exactly what they should do once the baby is born.

"I just want to hold it and see it. And you guys take a picture of it, right? Once you take the picture of it, that's all I think I need out of it," she says to Nancy and Nurse Carolyn. She read the booklets the hospital gave her, about how some parents like to dress the dead baby, and talk to it, and take a lot of pictures. She doesn't know for sure, says Julie, but she thinks she won't want to do all that.

"For me, I think that there's a point where . . . doing things with the baby when it's dead is like a little beyond reality to me, you know?"

Nancy Sullivan nods her head: yes, yes, yes.

"But holding it and seeing it is just what I think anybody would desire to do. Unless you were, you know, not confident enough that you could handle it. And who knows that till the time comes? But irregardless, I'll force myself to do it. 'Cause it seems like everyone's told me that you would regret it if you didn't. So I want to . . ."

"Okay," says Nancy.

"I don't have any more tears," she says, as much to herself as to Nancy. "I think they're all dried up. Well, right now!" The assemblage laughs gently, reassuringly. "There's always a fresh supply!"

"You keep saying, 'I'm strong-I'm strong-I'm strong!' But I *know* you're strong," says Nancy, taking Julie's hand in hers.

"I've cried my fair share," says Julie. There's a general murmuring among the women at the bedside.

"The strongest people cry a lot," someone says.

"I cried a lot this morning," says the woman in the bed.

"She did," the midwife tells the others. "She did cry a lot this morning, that's right!"

"It probably had something to do with the shock, the way I was waking up . . . "

Nancy Sullivan prepares to leave the room.

"I'll be back in a minute," she says.

1920: 7:20 P.M.

In the Intermediate Neonatal Care Unit, a plumpish, middle-aged volunteer wearing green scrubs holds tiny withdrawing crack addict Timothy Edwards, born Monday in the ambulance. She coos at him, tries to get the apathetic red-haired infant to suck on a bottle. In the dozen or so warming units in the three rooms, lie tiny babies, mostly preemies. One little girl named Tanya wears a Cabbage Patch doll dress (much cheaper than official preemie clothes) and makes small mewling sounds, like a new puppy that wants to nurse. A nurse approaches her warmer with a bottle, eyeing Tanya's monitor readings above.

In the coffee/supply room down the hall, three nurses talk about Julie Bouchard's patient, the sixteen-year-old who'd had a normal birth, yet died eight days later from an embolus because of having intercourse too early after her baby's birth. Becky Abramson shakes her head sadly as she dumps sauce, tomatoes, and onions onto a huge taco from the cafeteria in South Hospital. Carolyn Bachhuber eats a salad she brought. ("Five more pounds to go," she mutters grimly. "Just five more pounds.")

179

Nancy Sullivan drinks coffee and reads aloud from *People* magazine's report of "The Preppie Murder." Her own daughter, Megan, knew the victim. Another good reason for the Sullivans to have moved to Portland from New York, she says. Talk turns to how having children ruins your sex life. Well, says Nancy, at least once you've had kids, it'll never be the same again.

2030: 8:30 P.M.

Nurse-Midwife Nancy Sullivan takes a long, deep breath before entering the Special Delivery Room.

"I'm scared to deliver this baby," she says softly.

The lights in the room are turned down low, the kind of glow perfect for a romantic evening. On the windowsill, three yellow tulips bloom in a vase of clear glass. An epidural anesthetic has been put into the spine of Julie O'Brien, who is talking about whether young Joshua should come see the baby when all is over.

"They say that children won't put themselves through anything they can't handle," she says.

"Who says that?" snaps a voice from the far end of the room. "I just don't think he's old enough to make that decision!" Julie's mother, a small, glamorous blonde in an expensive nubby beige handknit sweater and matching linen slacks, has just arrived from D.C., where she lives with her third husband.

The population of the large Special Delivery Room is increasing. In addition to Annette and Lori, and Julie's mother, there is Maurice, very dark and clad in impeccably pressed chinos and a handknit pullover. An odd couple, Julie's boyfriend and her mother sit together, scant inches from touching. Soon to become a father for the third time, with a third woman, Maurice presses his spine into the back of the sofa and sighs heavily, frequently. His gaze is fixed upon the silent, manic television set suspended above, while the grandmother-to-be elaborately examines her beautifully red-lacquered fingernails.

Nurse Carolyn Bachhuber, a muscle twitching furiously in her left cheek, views the pair on the sofa. Taking it all in, she shoots sympathetic glances at her patient as she adjusts the fetal heart monitor strap on Julie's belly. From across the room, mother continues to hector daughter in tight, tense tones about the folly of involving small boys in large decisions.

It isn't, she tells Julie, as though the baby is *real* to Joshua.

"Yes, it is," Julie tells her mother in the voice of a tired parent. "He's been looking forward to having a little brother or sister, and has been feeling it move inside me."

"What? What!" It is a gurgling sound as, repelled, the older woman reels back, shuddering daintily. She exchanges a look with the dark man seated beside her. He shrugs, raising his glance back to the TV set. The silent picture shows three of *The Golden Girls* sitting at their kitchen table. Betty White is wearing a Girl Scout uniform with a sashful of merit badges.

Tears spill from Julie's eyes, and she dabs at them with a torn, ragged hankie as she continues to speak.

"I'll know how horrible it is for me, and I'm certainly not going to present him with something that, you know, is hard for me, too. I was just thinking that on the outside chance . . ." She takes in a big breath, and lets it out slowly. "The greatest hope is that it would be tiny, that its veins would be very noticeable, that it wouldn't have any hair. That we could wrap it in a blanket and put a hat on it, and he might just see it for a moment if it's, you know, visible. I mean, I'm not sold on the idea, so . . ." She looks to Nancy Sullivan, beseeching.

"Well, I think letting him see it is probably best," says the nurse-midwife. Julie's mother glares coldly, jealously, at this intruder, this person who isn't even a real doctor, for God's sake.

"You're worried about me seeing it," Julie states, looking directly at the midwife.

"Yeah," Nancy admits. "But I think you need to see it one way or another."

"Well, I don't expect this to be pleasant, but I think . . ." Her soft voice trails off.

"I know," says Nancy, "I know."

"Well," says Julie, her voice breaking, the tears beginning

181

again. "Well, that's why everybody's here, right?"

"Um-hmm," murmurs Nancy. "That's why everybody's here."

"We . . . I dealt with it as much as I can deal with it before it's happened, so . . . " The nurse-midwife nods her assent. "I'm as ready as I can be for something like this. There's no way that I can probably imagine the worst."

"Well, they say that usually you imagine the worst," interjects Nurse Carolyn Bachhuber.

" . . . and usually what you do is focus on all the normal things," says Nancy.

"Yes," agrees Julie. "And not spend too much time, and I won't . . . and I think I know myself to be a fairly emotional person who just won't really need to stare at it and keep it for a day or anything like that. So it's easier for me to just brush away an unpleasant memory or something." She is weeping aloud now.

"You," says Nancy, holding her hand again, "are going to be okay."

"I know. I know. But I've heard so many things from other women that went through this, that even though it was hard, real hard, they were glad they didn't miss the opportunity. And the women who had really felt bad that they hadn't held their babies. It made them feel guilty later, that they were *detached.*" She looks at the midwife. "I trust you, really, a lot," she says. "And I think if you tell me it's not a good idea to look at the baby, then I can deal with that."

"Okay," says Nancy.

"How's that sound?" Julie asks.

"Good," says the midwife.

"Okay," says the younger woman, trembling beneath her hospital gown. "Am I shaking because I'm scared, or cold and I don't know it, or what?"

Nurse Carolyn tells her that the epidural anesthesia can make you shake.

"Well," says Julie, calm and poise restored, "I think everybody ought to go out to dinner, have a glass of wine, and come back!"

Everyone laughs, the tension broken.

"The watched pot never boils," says Carolyn.

"I think," says Nancy Sullivan, "that I'll go take a little nap."

"Really?"

"Yeah."

"I'll let you," says Julie, smiling at her.

"I don't think I want to sleep, but I think I'll lie down."

"Okay," says the woman on the bed.

"I'll just be upstairs, lying down."

2126: 9:26 P.M.

Harriet Grackle is in the Exam Room. She thinks she is in labor. She is not, and as soon as a resident comes in, she will be told so.

Two bikers sit on uncomfortable chairs down the hall from Harriet. One is Harriet's husband, Animal Grackle. What's left of his long brown hair is pulled into a rough ponytail, and under his black leather vest is a Harley-Davidson T-shirt, also black: TEARING UP THE COMPETITION. The other man, shorter but with similar physique, sports a bright gold T-shirt announcing 4-WHEELERS EAT MORE BUSH.

Up the hall from the Exam Room where Harriet lies with splayed legs and crossed fingers, a handful of residents and nurses are gathered around the nurses' station: Residents Bob Hicks, Kathy Doyle and Linda Moore, and Nurses Carolyn Bachhuber and Becky Abramson. Hicks is telling a story about twins who were supposed to be already dead in utero, so great care wasn't expended on their behalf. Then they were born, squawking—and okay.

"You feel like, 'It's a miracle!'" says Hicks.

Cindy Shepard, a nurse visiting from the Mother-Baby Unit downstairs, counters with The Tale of the Phantom Twins. A woman came into L&D one night, claiming she had twins inside. She was from Longview, up in Washington, she said, and so had no records, and claimed she was in active labor. Turned out not to be pregnant at all.

The tales get worse. Nurse Becky tells of the very pregnant woman in the icy winter auto wreck who went straight through the windshield, which gave her a very efficient c-section. The mother died; the healthy newborn was found bawling lustily in the snow several feet away.

Someone else tells of the Oregon woman living in Texas who told everyone she was pregnant. Even fooled her husband. Then, at "term," she lay in wait for a genuinely pregnant woman, then gave her a fatal c-section with a car key. Tried checking herself into a hospital, claiming the baby was her own, self-delivered. It didn't work. She's in custody now while they try to figure out what to do with her. The dead woman's husband, with his new baby, another toddler and no wife, is a Mormon who says it's all God's Will.

2221: 10:21 P.M.

Julie O'Brien isn't feeling so hot. And with her epidural, she isn't feeling the urge to push, so she's being told when to bear down to help expel her baby. Her mother, who has migrated from the couch, is stationed now at the foot of the bed. Maurice has planted himself beside her, his head twisted back toward the mute television set, which displays a tall slinky blonde whose diamond necklace has apparently been stolen.

"I think," says Julie in a small, ghostly voice, "I'm going to be sick!"

"There's some little basins in that drawer," says Nurse Carolyn, gesturing to a cabinet on the other side of the bed. Women in labor often feel like vomiting, she assures her.

"How many more?" asks Julie.

"How many more pushes?" asks Nancy.

"Yeah. Maybe two?"

"Yeah . . . three or two."

"*Uuuuuh!* I don't think I can push anymore!"

"Yeah, it's hard," says Nancy.

"You," says Nurse Carolyn, "are doing a great job, Julie!"

Great job and all, Julie nonetheless moans.

"I can't do it anymore!"

"Almost there," says Carolyn.

Julie pants.

"Almost there," repeats the nurse.

Julie pants again.

"Doing great," whispers the nurse.

"Wonderful!" adds the nurse-midwife.

Julie pants and moans. Soft jazz plays on the radio. In the hallway outside, a telephone rings, unanswered. Julie makes a big grunting sound.

One more big push, and a baby is born.

Nurse-Midwife Nancy Sullivan assesses the newborn with professional eyes. The baby is about twelve inches long, weighs something under two pounds, probably. Two legs, two arms, and the customary number of fingers and toes, praise be! Head smaller than normal, but not so most people could tell the difference. Not much in the way of a chin. Ears aligned oddly, the tops about even with the nostrils, rather than with the eyes. Eyes large and slitty, "mongoloid"-looking, but Nancy doesn't believe the child has Down's syndrome. Nothing a mother couldn't love so far. The genitalia? It's a coin-flip. Those little puffs could be either testicles or a swollen vulva, and that little thing there *could* be a penis. Or it could be a largish clitoris. Looks mostly female, but only an autopsy is going to show for sure.

"Is it a boy?" asks Julie, fingers crisping, hands reaching toward her child.

"Nooooo . . . " says the midwife, looking carefully again at what has just emerged. She makes a quick decision, settling the question for the here and now.

"A girl," says Nancy. "It's a girl. And she's real little."

"She's got hair, Julie," says Annette. "She's got black hair."

"She's alive?" asks Julie. "She can't start breathing or anything?"

"She might try to take a few breaths," answers Nurse Carolyn, "but she's very small, very early."

"You ever deliver one that small?" Julie asks Nancy, who is carefully, so carefully, wrapping the infant in a warmed white flannel blanket printed with pink, blue, and yellow ducklings.

"No, I haven't," replies the midwife, smiling down at mother and newborn. "She's my smallest baby."

Outside, in the hall, the phone stops ringing. On the radio, a mournful saxophone plays "Spring Will Be a Little Late This Year."

"It's God's grace that this one is not alive," murmurs Annette.

"Tiny little girl," says Nancy, in almost a whisper.

"She looks real good," says Carolyn. "She looks like babies her age look like."

"She won't take a breath, huh?" asks Julie.

"She might," says Nancy.

"She might," echoes Carolyn. "She kind of moved her lips."

"She did move her lips," agrees Nancy.

"And her heart was beating. I could tell," adds Carolyn.

A nurse opens the door to tell Nancy that another patient of hers thinks she's ruptured her membranes. Turning her head, Nancy asks her to find out if she needs to come in for an evaluation.

"This is called vernix," explains the nurse-midwife, stroking the child's cheek, which is covered with a pasty white substance. "It's what's on the premature babies. It's kind of like cold cream that keeps them from getting dried out."

The sax wails on.

"Her name is Emily," says Julie.

"Hello, Emily," says Nancy in a sweet, full, compassionate voice. "She looks tinier than I thought she would."

"See her little fingers?" Julie asks dreamily.

"Has she started breathing?" someone asks.

"No," says Carolyn, "'cause she looks real early."

"See, I don't really think she's that early," says Nancy. "She just didn't grow."

"Yeah," agrees Carolyn, "'cause she should be almost thirty weeks."

"Yeah, that's what they were saying on the ultrasound. That's why they knew something was wrong," says Nancy. "Her body wasn't the right size."

"She's got long legs," observes Annette.

"Real long legs..." Julie strokes the baby's tiny hands with an index finger. "You know what's amazing, is when we were looking at the ultrasound, these look like the little fingerbones I saw on the ultrasound. Yet, I can't believe this has happened. I know what happened. I know everybody knows that..."

Joshua. What about Joshua?

"What did you decide about that?" asks Carolyn. "Did you want him to see her?"

Julie bites her lip, looking down intently at her tiny daughter. "Probably, with a gown on, and the cap, and with her face cleaned up, she probably wouldn't look so much worse than, not atrocious . . ."

"She doesn't look atrocious now," says a soft-voiced female alongside the bed.

"She's beautiful," says another, firmly.

"When you wash her, the stuff will come all off, but I bet her face won't get any pinker. It'll get bluer, right?" asks Julie.

"Well, I don't think she's going to live very long," says Nurse Carolyn, gently.

"I understand that," sighs Julie.

"Once she dies, they then all . . . look just gray," explains Carolyn.

"Well, why doesn't somebody just go get Josh?" suggests Julie. "We'll get him up here, and see what he decides to do. Call him." She looks down at her newborn. "She feels like a baby. She weighs enough to feel like a baby."

"Um-hmmm," Nancy affirms. "You did a great job."

"I did," says Julie.

"Yeah, you did what you had to do," says the nurse-midwife.

"I don't want to take the credit, though."

"You go right ahead," says Nancy, smiling.

Across the room, Annette is on the phone. "Your mom had the baby, and you can come down and look at her if you want."

"She might not be alive anymore," says Carolyn. "But she was when she was born."

"I could feel her heart beating," says Nancy. "Look at all the hair she has!"

"You don't want to see her?" Annette asks Joshua on the phone. "That's okay, Josh." She says good-bye, hangs up, returns to the bedside.

"Thanks, Annette. That was hard to do. He was pretty definite, huh? All the literature says the child would not put himself through anything he can't handle. So it's good he had an option."

187

"Oh, for heaven's sake, Julie," her mother says. "To let a little boy make such a decision!"

Maurice looks at the clock on the far wall, checking the time against his Rolex.

Nurse Carolyn Bachhuber puts her stethoscope to the baby's tiny chest.

"She's still alive," she announces. "Her heart is beating, but it's getting real slow."

"What shall I do with her?" asks Julie, panic suddenly in tear-filled eyes.

"Just hold her real tight," advises the nurse-midwife. "She likes being close to her mother. It's the only place she's ever been."

Maurice, who has been rocking back and forth on feet shod in silvery-gray Italian leather, plucks a piece of lint from his beautiful sweater. The bit of fluff floats, unnoticed, from dark fingers to the beige vinyl tile floor.

"Little Emily! She looks like she would've been so perfect," croons Julie O'Brien, holding the small bundle to her chest.

"Yeah, she does," says Nancy. "She has beautiful features!"

"She has really big eyes," adds Carolyn.

"She's got a really pretty mouth. Pretty mouths kind of run in my family, don't they?" Julie asks, looking down the bed at her silent mother, who has spoken only once since her granddaughter was born. With effort, the woman twists her own pretty mouth into a small smile.

"Well, we're just going to do this till she's gone, I guess," says Julie. "Till we're sure she's no longer alive."

Through it all, Nurse-Midwife Nancy Sullivan is keeping a sharp eye out for the essential, telling details: Is the patient bleeding too much? Are the drapes properly placed? What about her blood pressure?

"You going to let me have this placenta?" asks Nancy.

"Shall I push?"

"Sure—if you're ready," says Carolyn. "She's been a perfect patient, hasn't she?"

"She sure has!" says Nancy.

Palpating for a contraction, Nurse Carolyn hurts Julie.

"Owww!"

"Sorry!"

"I'll just take it out of your five-cent tip!"

"I thought I got a dime," replies the nurse. Laughter, then silence, except for "I Remember April" on the radio.

"It's not like you can manipulate her much," says Julie. "Her little back feels like it's so bony, and her bones ... she is so skinny! But her head is so heavy. I can't believe it. Her head feels like it weighs two pounds! You don't even have to have her up against your body to hold her body, because your hands just kind of hold her by themselves."

Everyone chimes in with admiration for this new person:

"Look at that, her pointed upper lip!"

"You would have looked good in Max Factor, honey!"

"She would've looked good in anything!"

"And would've raised an eyebrow or two!"

"Come on, Emily," joshes Julie. "You're being put to the test to see if your genes are stronger on my side or not!"

"She's pretty brown, Julie," says freckly blond Lori, herself the mother of two mixed children. "From the beginning—and they get darker!"

"Oh, little legs," exclaims Julie. "Look how she's got her little legs tucked up underneath her!"

"Her eyes! She's got the hugest eyes!" This from Lori.

"Well, they're probably real swollen," says Julie.

"Yeah," says Nancy, "they are. They're real swollen eyes."

"They would've been real big eyes, though," insists Julie.

Lori turns to Maurice, silent at the foot of the bed.

"That makes three girls in a row for you," she says. "You're just a real girl-maker! The man determines the sex, you know. Well, you make beautiful girls."

"Great," he says in a deep baritone, making a small, ironic bow to the assembled women. "Thank you." Despite the jaunty gesture, Maurice looks profoundly ill. As if he'd rather be someplace else, anyplace else, on earth right now.

"Are you going to take a picture? Do you want to wash the baby?" asks Julie.

"Well, I just hate to put her through that when"—the nurse hesitates—"when she's still ... "

"When she's still breathing?" Julie finishes for her.

"Long toes," observes Lori, fair head craned over the baby. "You have long toes, Maurice?"

"Uh...she didn't get anything long from me! Unless she would've been long-winded!"

There's kindly laughter for this.

"As unpleasant as it may have been for you guys to be here, I appreciate it," says Julie, her glance taking in everyone. "Each and every one of you that are here, I appreciate it."

"She just gets to walk the streets of gold sooner," says Lori, looking at the infant's still form.

"They're waiting for her at the Pearly Gates," echoes Annette.

"She doesn't have to deal with all the suffering in this world," says Lori.

"She never has to be a teenager," Annette says.

"She never has to be *my* teenager," says Julie, laughing. "That's where the saving grace came in for this child. Poor Emily!"

Silence again, but for Ol' Blue Eyes singing "My Way" on KMHD.

"Well, guess what?" says Julie. "Over there somewhere, and I don't know what we did with it, but somebody has to put a little bracelet on her. It's by the window, I think."

In silent ceremony, a tiny gold bracelet is placed on the infant's right hand.

"Boy, she's cold. Very cold," says Julie. "Not a good sign, huh?"

"She's cold," agrees Nancy.

"Real cold," repeats Julie.

"She's so darling," says Annette. "I can't believe it."

"Let's put some nice pink clothes on this little mixed child," says Julie. "So they can recognize her African roots when she gets there. Let's dedicate her."

"Dedicate her to God?" asks Nancy.

"Yeah, that's what we do at New Song Church," explains Lori.

"Would you like to lead the prayer?" Julie asks her friend, then changes her mind. "No, let's let Maurice lead the prayer."

190

Glancing again at the wall clock, Maurice sighs, then begins:

"Father, in Jesus' name we thank you, Lord, for your goodness and your mercy that endures forever. Thank you, Lord, because you love us like we are, that you love us too much to leave us the way we are. We pray God that you will take this child now, and that you would welcome her into . . . " He stumbles, then recovers. "Uh . . . into Heaven. That you would cause each one of us to not be forgetful of this event, of this time, of life, what it's all about."

"Um-hmmm," comes a general murmur from the small congregation.

"Help us to live it to the fullest. Help us to live our lives that we might glorify you. We say unto you, in Jesus' name, amen."

Silence. More Sinatra from the radio.

Julie smiles at her daughter.

"Emily, as much as I love you, I'm not going to kiss your gooey face!"

Again, laughter. She holds the baby toward the nurse.

"Well, why don't you check her one more time for vital signs, just to be sure before I give her up. Do you mind, Carolyn? I guess it's a pretty good sign if her arm's cold?"

Carolyn can't detect a heartbeat.

"What do you do with her from here, immediately? Just clean her up, and put a gown on her?"

"We weigh her and measure her," says Carolyn. "We do footprints, and take a picture for you. You want the prints, don't you?"

"Not necessarily," says Julie.

"We do them, and then if you want them, you can have them," says Carolyn with a small shrug.

"Okay."

"And then a picture."

"Joshua said tonight he wanted pictures," says Annette.

"Okay," says Julie. Her mother, still fixed at the end of the bed, casts her eyes heavenward, but says nothing.

"And then we just put her name on her, and that's pretty much all," Carolyn finishes.

"Okay. Okay."

"And then if she goes downstairs, if you want her to . . . where they, uh, keep them. We'll have her in the back for a little while, if you want to see her before she goes."

"Did you want to be alone with her for a little while?" asks Nancy.

"No," replies Julie, smiling. "I've had eight months alone with her. It was just nice to be able to share her. You can take her."

Tenderly, oh so tenderly, Julie surrenders the dead child to Nancy Sullivan. Then, leaning back on her pillow, she looks at her baby for one last moment, then from the midwife to the nurse, to Maurice, to her two friends. Finally, Julie's gaze travels to the face of her pursed-lipped mother, whose mascara looks like it might be smudged, just a little.

On the radio, Frank Sinatra is singing "Teach Me Tonight."

CHAPTER THIRTEEN

DAY 7: Sunday, April 17

("Give her kisses! Give her kisses!"
says the mother, age thirty-eight.)

THERE'S A LOT OF curiosity about thirty-year-old First-Year Resident Gary Hoffman, both on 4NE and down in the Mother-Baby Unit. Not that he's a particularly mysterious person. It probably just has something to do with L&D's general habit of not prying into the lives of patients, of not offering too much about yourself right away. The ships-that-pass-in-the-night business becomes such a part of surviving in a job that's life and death, thirty-six hours of it at a whack. L&D: Labor and Delivery. L&D: Life and Death. Sometimes it just spills over into the relationships between the residents and the nurses. Over a four-year OB/GYN residency, you find out a lot about each other. But this is Gary's first year, so there's still that curiosity.

Looking at Gary Hoffman, you'd think he's led a charmed life. Toward the tail end of a thirty-six-hour shift, his eyes might be red-rimmed, but that's all that shows of the exhaustion he feels sucking at his bones. If anything, he looks even more handsome tired, with the glossy dark wavy hair, the Tom Selleck moustache, the Cary Grant cleft in the chin. (This, thinks more than one female doctor, projects a nurse or two, is a man whom the years are only going to improve. And such a nice guy, to boot. How *is* that cloning research coming along, anyway?)

The resident seems unflappable, the essence of equanimity. He probably doesn't even guess he's called DDH—Darling Doctor Hoffman—behind his back. He just steps aside nimbly when palsied Debbie Pellegrini down in MBU bobbles from her wheelchair in the direction of his crotch. Most women aren't that direct.

SHIT HAPPENS.

Dr. Hoffman saw that bumper sticker not long ago, and he wants one. Put it up in the garage, maybe.

A quick résumé wouldn't show anything too special. Gary Hoffman: second of five kids, father a business manager for an electronics firm, mother a teacher working for years with special-ed and retarded kids and now teaching fourth grade. Grew up in Massachusetts, went to the University of Maine. Majored in biology, thinking maybe he'd do research. But the lab work, the bench work, it wasn't for him. Married Ericka Weiss, who came to the university on an exchange program from Portland. Becoming a doctor seemed like a good idea; got accepted at St. Louis University Medical School.

Almost right away, Gary Hoffman knew that delivering babies was where it was at for him. It's fun. You have healthy— well, for the most part, healthy—patients. It's a happy time, you know? It's a really good feeling when you can deliver a baby, a nice baby, to some nice parents. But up here, there's lots of times when you deliver babies and it's like: *God! What's going to happen to this poor child?*

Like the first patient Gary ever had here as an intern. It was less than a year ago that he walked into that room. The mother's in active labor, screaming uncontrollably. On the left-hand side of the bed is this young guy—seventeen, eighteen maybe—who's her current boyfriend. And on the other side of the bed is a forty-five-year-old Hell's Angel. They're both there because nobody knows which one is the father, just screaming and yelling at each other.

And they're yelling at the laboring woman because she's making too much noise. Then they start yelling at each other again because one of them says this baby's taking too long, and the baby's going to get a licking when it gets out for taking too long!

Gary's examining the woman, and scared to death, you know, it being his first delivery ever. Those are the worst ones, where you think: *This poor kid!* Like being born with three strikes against him already! But it comes with the territory.

It has nothing to do with the patients here, most of them anyway, being poor. As far as Dr. Gary Hoffman is concerned, he won't turn his back on anybody. But that malpractice stuff is awful. Some patients are really threatening. He doesn't think he has to deal with that. Like if you go get your car fixed, you don't tell the mechanic, "Now, I want this done, and I want this done, and I want this done. And if you don't do that, I'm gonna *sue* you!" He doesn't want to take care of those patients, the obviously sue-happy ones. He'll just say, "I don't think I can do a good job of taking care of you." Let them go somewhere else.

Fetal demise, babies dying, that has to be the worst part of being an obstetrician. Nobody's guaranteed a perfect baby. Never, never, never. There are no guarantees. That's just life. There's nothing you can do about it. People don't realize it, people who haven't lost children. People who have not dealt with death. People come in to have a baby, you know, and not a lot of people think about driving home with an empty new car seat, having to go home to the baby's room that they've fixed up, to that empty, mocking crib. *Here's your baby's room, and it's empty!* When it happens in the hospital, it really hits Dr. Gary Hoffman hard, because it brings back the worst possible time in his life. The time when his own daughter died.

His firstborn, his beautiful Alexandra.

SHIT HAPPENS, oh yes, it happens. Like Alexandra, beautiful gorgeous beloved wonderful miraculous Alexandra, born at the beginning of Gary's second year of med school. And then dead one day in her crib, gone forever. SIDS, Sudden Infant Death Syndrome. Never to be older than sixteen months. People think it only happens in the first few months of life, but they're wrong. Usually, it does. But Alex was among the 2 percent of SIDS babies who die after a year. She lived a full sixteen months, oh yes.

Never was there such a child: Never will there be such a

child again. She was so full of energy, so full of life. Gary and Ericka were both constantly amazed, every day. The day before it happened, the little family had been playing together. They have some incredible pictures of her. Alex lived her whole life in sixteen months, that's what it comes down to. And they brought her out here to bury her, another reason to come to OHSU for the residency. Another reason to stay in Portland.

Ericka and Gary weren't really trying to have another baby, not right away anyway, but they had begun talking about it before Alex died. Cassandra is beautiful, almost six months old now. She's gorgeous, too, a lot like Alex, but in other ways really different. Originally, their plan was for four kids. Now they're not sure.

Kids are so precious. They really give you something to live for. Ericka, there's one thing that really kills her, she even cries sometimes when they're out, say, in a supermarket. She'll see some mother, with the little kid reaching out to grab something—they don't know better, that's just what kids do!—and the mother slaps the kid. Ohh! It hurts so bad, it hurts so bad it's *terrible*!

After his four years of residency, Gary Hoffman would like to do a subspecialty. But that's another three years of a fellowship, another three years of delayed gratification. By the time you start college and go four years and then do four years of med school and four years of residency, you've gone from first to twelfth grade again. Twenty-four years total. A long time. And the debt is incredible. Gary Hoffman owes about $40,000, $45,000. Some of his classmates owe more than $100,000.

1554: 3:54 P.M

An overcast Sunday afternoon, looks like it might rain. Dr. Gary Hoffman looks over The Board. Things are slow, with four empty rooms.

Dr. Hoffman smiles as he thinks of Harriet Grackle, one of his favorite-ever clinic patients. From a phone call he just took, the resident knows she is, as he smiles, zooming toward

Marquam Hill with her husband on the Harley, semiconvinced she's in labor. Even though he's fairly certain there won't be a little Grackle hatched tonight, the resident looks forward to visiting with the couple.

In Room 18, Tamara Horton, twenty-one-years old, thirty-four weeks along, believes she is in labor. She is being sent down to the Mother-Baby Unit on the third floor.

Marcia Frampton, the thirty-eight-year-old laboring in Room 8, is, like her sister accompanying her this afternoon, a private patient of Dr. Mark Nichols.

In Room 2, Elizabeth Duncan is clearly in pain, but just makes loud sighs as large tears roll down her cheeks.

Special Delivery is where the action is this afternoon. That's where Pearl Monley is, sick and tired of pushing to get that kid out. Pearl, a twenty-five-year-old black woman with long, long hair, holds hands with her boyfriend, Clarence, the father of her other child as well as this one. Her notation on The Board says she's had "minimal prenatal care" at Grace Peck Clinic. But no drugs. ("Uh-uh! No *way*!")

In the room with the couple are Dr. Gary Hoffman, medical student Anina Merrill, Nursing Student Deona Koth, and Nurse Carolyn Bachhuber.

The television set offers a tough-looking gent in cowboy garb. ("She's been raped and murdered by those fiends!" he announces fiercely to other tough-looking gents.)

On the bed, Pearl curls up her red-nailed toes and, chomping on gum as she grimaces, issues a warning of her own: "Okay! You guys ready?"

Yes. Yes, we're ready, nurse, doctor, students, and boyfriend all assure the laboring woman.

"I wanna have a baby, you guys!" Sweat glistens on her dark brow.

"We *want* you to have a baby," says Nurse Carolyn Bachhuber, grinning. "Do you feel like pushing now?"

The woman on the bed sighs heavily. They just don't seem to understand!

"*I keep trying to tell you guys! I'm tired, and to push takes a little strength, you know?*"

We know, we know, the group assures her.

"Pearl! Pearl, listen," says Dr. Hoffman, leaning closer to

her head, looking straight into her eyes. "You're doing a *good* job!"

Another push.

Dr. Hoffman inserts the second and third fingers into Pearl's vagina, helping to stretch the perineum. She isn't going to need an episiotomy, he decides.

Another push. Then another.

"*Uuuuunh!*" Pearl grunts. This is hard work, very damned hard work!

"*Aaaaagh!*"

Finally, a big push, and a baby is born.

"A little boy!" exults the handsome doctor with the cleft in his chin.

"Is he okay?" asks the mother. "Is he okay?"

"Is he *okay!*" answers Dr. Hoffman. Pearl and Clarence's son is fine and dandy, his umbilical cord looped into what is called a "true knot." The resident begins to palpate Pearl's abdomen, encouraging the placenta to be expelled.

"*Ewwwwww! Oh, yecch!*" says Pearl. "*Eeeeeh!*" she screams. "Are you trying to *pull* it or something?"

1820: 6:20 P.M.

Frannie Fenner and her husband, Ronnie, enter Room 16. Frannie—cute and cheery, a freckled blonde clad in a peach-colored velour running suit, is eighteen, and this is her first baby. Though she is small in build, her belly is enormous. Ronnie holds her hand. He's wearing the Oregon Man's off-work uniform: faded blue jeans and worn Nikes, his denim jacket, its once-white fleece lining grubby and gray, worn over the obligatory plaid flannel shirt.

Nursing Student Deona Koth does the intake.

"Any problems with this pregnancy?" she asks the young couple.

"Only that it won't come out!" replies the teenager. "He is one stubborn little boy. I've had—what, Ronnie, two or three ultrasounds?—and we know it's a little boy."

The couple laugh easily together.

"We've tried everything," Frannie continues. *"Candy! There's candy out here! And toys!"*

At forty-two weeks along, two weeks *overdue*, Frannie has, at the suggestion of her doctor at Pill Hill's prenatal clinic, come in to have labor induced.

No, she hasn't been using alcohol. No, no street drugs.

"Are you kidding? *Frannie?* That'll be the day!" says her husband, rolling his eyes. He is nineteen.

Deona makes notes on the chart, then the nursing student begins strapping the fetal heart monitor around Frannie Fenner's belly.

In Room 8, a haggard-looking Joan Baez is being interviewed by a ponderous Ed Bradley on *60 Minutes*.

On the bed a few feet away, Marcia Frampton, her long, frizzy dark curls tangled on the pillow, moans with a contraction. She turns her head toward her doctor.

"I'm in so much pain, Dr. Nichols!"

"I know," says her obstetrician. "I know. We're going to do something about that soon." Dr. Nichols has asked for an epidural for his patient.

In the hall outside, the laboring woman's sister sits with Marcia's little three-year-old daughter. Stacy has inherited her mother's dark eyebrows, beneath which huge damp brown eyes glower. Despite the warmth of the hallway, the child insists upon wearing her ruffled lavender jacket. The small girl curls in a fetal position on her aunt's lap, sucking the thumb of one hand while she fondles a tiny heart-shaped pierced earring with her other hand.

"I want my *mommy!*" she whimpers. "Why can't I be with my *mommy?*" She wipes her runny nose along the sleeve of the lavender jacket.

Stacy Frampton is one of the rare ones in late-twentieth-century America, a preschooler whose mother chooses to stay home full time with her young children—and can afford to. Doug and Marcia had definite ideas about that from the start, ten years ago, when they married. Both came from large families. Doug's mother stayed home with her six children, and Marcia, who had four brothers and sisters, always wished her

199

widowed mother had been able to. She and Doug met at Reed College, in the fall of their freshman year, and just knew they were meant for each other, the short, plump, red-haired young man and the tall, dark, and graceful stalk of a young woman. Friends teased them, calling them "Mutt and Jeff," but they knew.

After graduating (Doug with a degree in math, Marcia with a B.A. degree in art, with a specialty in painting), they backpacked all over Europe, lived together for a couple of years, then married when both were twenty-eight. The plan was that they would wait five years, working and putting together some money for a down payment on a house, before starting their family. Doug and a couple of other former Reedies started a computer software firm, and Marcia got a job in the office of an art gallery.

Five years into the marriage, Marcia went off the pill. Expecting to be pregnant the next month. No such luck, either that month or the next or the next or the next. For a year, each worried separately, silently, that there was perhaps some sort of perverse divine retribution here, punishment for the abortion Marcia had during their sophomore year.

Then Marcia heard from someone in her weekly quilting group about the fertility clinic on Pill Hill. She didn't think she was ready for that, but another quilter, a woman who had never had any trouble, said Dr. Mark Nichols, her OB/GYN on The Hill, was marvelous.

So Marcia started coming to The Hill to see Dr. Nichols, and liked him so much she talked her sister Jacqui into switching to him. They were both glad they did. They can't believe how people are so prejudiced against coming to Pill Hill to have their babies, how they yammer on and on about they "deserve" to go someplace like Good Samaritan or St. Vincent's or Emanuel, with their hotel atmosphere and fancy-shmancy meals. Or that they don't want to be around minority women, or women who use drugs during pregnancy. As though they're going to catch a crack-smoking habit from them! (Usually, they're slurping up a glass of wine while they bitch about this.) Well, Marcia would go anywhere Dr. Nichols was delivering babies. She's having a baby, for Christ's sake, not throwing a cocktail party!

Once she started coming to Dr. Nichols, things happened. He set her up for a diagnostic laparoscopy. While she was under general anesthesia, he was able to look into her fallopian tubes. Turned out there was an obstruction, a little scar tissue or something, and Dr. Nichols cleared it out. It was that simple. Two weeks post-op, Marcia was pregnant. Twice she got pregnant, and twice she miscarried—the second one in the sixth month. People can be just awful about that, acting as though you haven't lost a live person. But Dr. Nichols was wonderful.

Marcia heard somewhere that Dr. Nichols and his wife lost a baby once. But she'd never presume to ask him about it, anymore than she'd presume to call him Mark. There is something reassuring about the traditional behavior of the doctor-patient relationship, something appealing about the formality. One thing she liked right away about Dr. Nichols was that during her first visit with him, rather than immediately calling her Marcia, he asked her what she preferred to be called. Nice.

The third time was the charm. When Marcia was pregnant for four months with Stacy, she knew this one was a keeper. She didn't have more than three or four weeks of morning sickness, and she kept on working at the gallery until the beginning of her eighth month. And then, she quit just so she could nest—get the curtains for the baby's room finished, and stitch the binding around the edges of the crib quilt she had started three years back. Stacy came out perfect, fine, with Marcia's dark hair and eyebrows so heavy they nicknamed her "Groucho" for a couple of months. (Until everyone was doing it, and they realized the poor kid was going to hate them for it later!)

There was another miscarriage, about a year or so after Stacy's birth. But somehow that wasn't as heartbreaking as the earlier ones. And this pregnancy hasn't given her one bit of trouble.

The door to Room 8 opens, and Anesthesiology Resident Robert Goldman comes in.

"I'm here to give Mrs. Frampton her epidural," he announces. "Would you mind waiting outside?"

"No, no—that's fine," answers Doug Frampton, rising from his chair.

"You are *one welcome sight*!" Marcia tells the anesthesiologist. She turns to her husband. "Honey, you look like you could use a cup of coffee. Why don't you and Jacqui go down to the cafeteria and get Stacy some kind of little treat?"

"I thought you'd never ask," jokes her husband. "See you in a few minutes."

Dr. Goldman asks Marcia to roll onto her left side.

"This is going to be cold and wet," he tells her, beginning to smear the Betadine in a circle on her back.

"You weren't kidding!" responds Marcia.

As the resident swabs the center of the bright orange Betadined circle with alcohol-soaked pads, Nurse Becky Abramson holds Marcia's hand. Dr. Goldman next injects lidocaine to numb the area. Despite her resolve to remain still, the patient jerks and yelps.

"Now we need you to arch your back," instructs Dr. Goldman.

Marcia Frampton grips the nurse's hand with her own strong right hand, its middle finger calloused from years of meticulous quilting.

"I'm ready," she says through gritted teeth.

"It's not going to be *that* bad," says the nurse, laughing.

"The hell you say," Marcia replies good-naturedly. "Don't forget I've *done* this before!" Her teeth stay clenched.

Dr. Goldman skillfully slips the needle into her spine.

"*Jeeez-us!* Oh, Christ on a cracker! I hate this part!" says Marcia.

No reply from the intent anesthesiologist, who is threading in the anesthetic. At last, he is done.

"You are going to feel much better. Very soon," he promises, gathering up his equipment before exiting Room 8.

Marcia Frampton is going to feel much better. Very soon.

In administering an epidural anesthetic to a laboring woman, the doctor needs to do two things. One is to place an epidural catheter, a small plastic tube, in near the spine, high enough so that it will reach those nerves that travel from the lower part of the midbody, the ones that *innervate* the uterus, and will aid in relieving the pain of labor's early first stage.

However, during the second stage of labor, the anesthesiologist also needs to be able to give an anesthetic that will sink down into the lower parts of the spinal cord, to numb the lower neural pathways along which travels the often-excruciating pain associated with labor's second stage.

Once labor has progressed, the cervix dilates, the baby's head starts to come down, and all the soft tissues of the mother's vagina and pelvis become stretched. In the second, "active," part of labor, a different route of nerves innervate the structures, causing a different feeling of pain. During this second stage of labor, these pain routes emerge much lower in the spine. They descend and sweep up and around, enervating the outside of the labia, the perineum, the vagina, and possibly the lower part of the cervix.

For a woman in labor, there are two main pathways involved in perceiving pain. First, there's the uterus itself. The body of the uterus is innervate, that is, there are nerves connected to it that emerge at the lower end of the thoracic part of the spinal cord. These nerves go down inside the abdominal cavity and sweep back up to innervate the uterus. In the early stages of labor, the sensory pain pathways come into the spinal cord, relatively high up at the lower part of the thorax, that part of the body which lies between the neck and abdomen.

The anatomy of the spinal cord is relatively simple. The vertebrae are star-shaped, with a circular base. Within a vertebra is a hollow area where the spinal cord resides. There are three bony projections off the back part of the vertebrae. In between the bases of the vertebrae lie pulpy disks. If the anesthesiologist gets the angle right, a needle can be inserted past the spine into the inner space. The spinal cord has a coating wrapped around it. This is the *dura*, which holds the spinal fluid around the cord.

In trying to place an anesthetic for a laboring woman's pain relief, the anesthesiologist has two choices. With a *spinal*, a needle is poked in past the bones, past the ligaments and tendons, through the surrounding dura into the spinal-cord space, getting spinal fluid to come back out. A small dose of anesthetic can thus be diffused relatively quickly, getting a strong block that shuts off sensory perception, as well as anesthetizing some of the motor pathways. The lower part of the woman's body is not only anesthetized against pain, it is also temporarily paralyzed.

With an *epidural,* which is the second way to give pain relief to a laboring woman, the needle is poked in past all the bony protuberances, past the ligaments, just inside the ligaments, but it does not pass through the dura. In this way, spinal fluid doesn't leak out. If the needle is in the epidural space—the space outside the dura—you can then inject a spinal anesthetic, numbing the nerves outside the spinal cord and diffusing down it, as well as blocking the nerve routes as they emerge from the spine and head out into the body. This method is somewhat safer to use when higher doses are injected, because they don't get so near the spinal cord. Another advantage of doing an epidural, rather than a spinal, is that, if placed right, the epidural does a good job of blocking sensory pathways, yet the mother is often left with some motor functions and is able to move her legs and still have a little bit of mobility in her labor bed.

However, in semi-emergency, or even crash, cesarean sections, a spinal—with its immediate effect—may be necessary, since an epidural takes a number of minutes to come on and give relief.

The anesthetic used in an epidural is basically the same type a dentist uses when extracting a tooth. Usually, it's an infusion of a member of the lidocaine family. Sometimes a small amount of narcotic is injected with it.

There are two ways to do an epidural. Generally, the patient lies on her side, back curved. A nurse holds her, wrapping an arm around her head, the other arm around her legs, bringing the mother's head toward her knees in an exaggerated fetal position. This bends the back outward, opening up the spiny projections, allowing a pathway for a needle to pass through.

Sometimes, if a woman has a curved spine, or because of obesity or other reasons, the spine's landmarks can't easily be found, and the mother must sit up, then bend over forward to spread the bony protuberances so that the anesthesiologist can poke around her back, in order to guide the needle in.

This way is harder on the baby because it compresses the fetal blood supply. Often, the choice is made *not* to give a woman an epidural if her physical anomalies seem to make this procedure dangerous.

Many a woman in the throes of an agonizing labor would be thrilled to lose all sensation, *period,* envying her grandmother, whose birthings all occurred while she was completely out, under general anesthesia. However, it's important to keep the muscle tone intact during early labor. As the baby's head comes down through the pelvis transverse, side to side, it needs to turn and proceed along its way, facing either down or up. Good muscle tone in the pelvis helps the head rotate to the anterior or posterior direction. Relax that region too soon, and the baby's head gets wedged in, and is continuously transverse.

As the baby's arrival nears, an additional dose of anesthetic can be given to the lower pelvic region, effectively numbing the perineal area between outer vagina and anus, and delivery is accomplished. Sometimes, if a woman gets too numb, the nurse (in consultation with the anesthesiologist) will dial the amount of the dose up or down to the right level, allowing the labor to progress in a good fashion.

It's all in the touch, the art of placing an epidural. It takes skill and experience, steely calm, and, perhaps, a certain personal detachment to pass a several-inch-long needle in through the skin, past the bones, past the ligaments. You have to have a good sense of where you're going, where those landmarks are. Poke around willy-nilly just getting the needle in, bump into too many bones, and it can be extremely painful for the woman—who hardly finds the process a delight to start with. Once the needle is in, once you pop past the ligaments, you can test whether you're in the epidural space by pushing with a connected, air-filled syringe. Keep pressing on the syringe, and once you've passed into the epidural space and lose some resistance, you've hit the bull's-eye. Go in too far, through the dura, and when you take the syringe off the needle there'll be spinal fluid dripping out. With this "wet tap," the woman may indeed have excellent pain relief, but the loss of spinal fluid is going to give her one hellacious headache, postdelivery.

1950: 7:50 P.M.

A half dozen residents and nurses sit and stand around the coffee/supply room, eating huge slabs of pizza. Extra cheese. Extra-thick crust. They're comparing the labor sounds different ethnic women make.

Hispanic women, Nurse Jeanne Gates reminds them, are very stoic, and under the worst pressure will call out: "*Ay-ay-ay-ay-ay!*"

Southeast Asian women, observes Chief Resident Kathleen Kennedy, hardly make a peep.

"Instead, they come in and shyly announce, 'Baby coming!' You'd think they were only two centimeters, then you check them and it'll practically be on the perineum!"

Early on, say the doctors, they learned to figure out how dilated a woman's cervix is by using their fingers. "And you get accurate at it," says Kathy Kennedy, telling the story of friends who needed to know how big a hole in their door was, in order to get a new lock for it.

"'Hey, simple,' I told 'em, and I just stuck my fingers in it. 'Four centimeters!' I told 'em. And it was!"

Outside the room, on the counter in front of the nurses' station, someone's Sharp Q727 tape deck plays Van Morrison's "Higher Than the World" tape.

2020: 8:20 P.M.

Marcia Frampton, in labor for nine hours, lies exhausted on her bed in Room 8. Her sister has gone, taking three-year-old Stacy home with her. Doug, Marcia's computer software designer husband, at five feet six inches a good four inches shorter than Marcia, is splayed out on the armchair beside her bed. Though not really focused, his eyes are turned to *Murder, She Wrote* on the television set above. Angela Lansbury's Jessica Fletcher is masquerading as someone else in order to investigate a friend's sister's murder.

"My God, doesn't that woman *ever* sit in front of a typewriter?" he says suddenly. "Every writer I've ever heard of has to spend *some* time alone in a room to get published, let alone be that famous!"

"What, Doug?" Marcia looks over toward her husband.

"Oh, nothing, honey. I just wish this kid would come out to meet us."

The fetal heart monitor is showing deep variables in the baby's heart rate, and with Marcia's epidural anesthesia affecting her ability to feel the contractions, compounded by simple exhaustion, she doesn't think she can push one more time. Dr. Nichols has decided to use the vacuum extractor.

"This makes me really nervous," says Marcia.

"Don't, worry," says Dr. Nichols. "It's going to be just fine!"

Doug Frampton, smiling tightly, stands alongside the bed, holding his wife's hand.

Dr. Nichols places the Mityvac into Marcia's vagina, against the baby's head. Then he applies the suction. With an unsettling resemblance to vacuuming out a doll from under the sofa, the child is pulled from inside her mother.

The little girl's cord, like that of Pearl Monley's son born three hours earlier, is configured in a true knot. Swaddled in warm flannel blankets adorned with baby animals printed in bright pastels, the newborn is carried down the hall to INCU, where her Apgar score is calculated at between 7 and 8.

On the bed in Room 8, Marcia begins to shudder and shake, reacting to the epidural anesthesia she received. As her husband starts out the door to follow the baby, the exhausted woman calls out to him.

"Give her kisses!" she shouts, her voice surprising in its vibrance.

"Give her kisses!"

In the nursery, Timothy Edwards, tiny and red-haired, sleeps as his mother, Cammie, stands over the warmer, watching his twitchy withdrawal from the crack she smoked just before he was born in the ambulance last Monday, six days ago. Standing beside Cammie is a once-pretty woman, now drained-looking, old for her forty or forty-five years. Tense, tired, and perhaps a little bit angry, she views her daughter's most recent gift to her. A sweet little thing, he is.

There are two more of Cammie's children at home: a two-year-old girl and a three-and-a-half-year-old boy. Timothy's grandmother has learned that the Children's Services Division wants to take this one from the hospital and put him straight into foster care. They're petitioning the court for immediate termination of Cammie's parental rights. If they do that, her new grandson will be adopted out.

The older woman sighs, a loud sound that attracts curious glances from halfway across the room, from the resident and the nurse examining Marcia Frampton's new baby.

She'll just have to adopt Timothy, too, no two ways about it. He can't be given away to strangers like that, like some mongrel puppy pawned off on strangers in a supermarket parking lot. The papers should be ready for them to pick up at the courthouse tomorrow. She just wishes Cammie would get her act together. Or if she isn't going to get her act together, if she isn't going to stop using those filthy drugs, if she isn't going to stop living on the streets when she's got a perfectly good room at home, then at least she should stop having these pitiful little messed-up babies, these broken little dolls someone else has got to try gluing back together.

Cammie Edwards just stares at the sleeping child and smiles. If she's thinking at all, which is doubtful, she's thinking that her boyfriend will probably bring her something good tonight.

Marcia Frampton's new daughter, being poked and prodded, howls from across the room.

2159: 9:59 P.M.

Elizabeth Duncan has been in the hospital since early this morning, and here it is almost ten at night. She is twenty-four, a secretary with a big insurance company, and has one child—plus a number of miscarriages, six or seven, Elizabeth can't remember.

Right now, Elizabeth is worried. She's worried that this baby won't come out alive. Or, worse, that it'll come out and then die in a week or a month or a year. She is worried that her small husband, who is from Mexico and who married her

208

two years ago because she was pregnant with a baby that didn't make it, is going to leave her if this baby doesn't live. She is worried that he'll leave her anyway because she's so big and fat. She is worried that he doesn't love her, because he is just sitting in his chair there, four feet away, when probably all the other husbands in all the other labor rooms are holding their wives, exhorting them to "*Breathe! Breathe! Breathe!*"

So Elizabeth Duncan is being very stoic about all the pain she's feeling, wiping away her silent tears and runny nose with a Kleenex wadded up in her right fist. When Dr. Gary Hoffman asks about her pain, she just answers "yes" or "no."

On the television set, the credits are rolling for *Married . . . With Children*, which, as far as Elizabeth could make out without actually watching it, had something to do with the husband making a mess of the house while trying to catch a mouse.

2208: 10:08 P.M.

It's very quiet. Frannie Fenner, the eighteen-year-old offering candy to her stubborn in utero child, has been sent down to the Mother-Baby Unit to begin induction. The Board is nearly empty. There's the weeping blond woman in Room 2, and in Room 10, Joni Phillips—the small, dark, unpleasant asthmatic woman still insisting she wants a tubal ligation after her delivery.

In Special Delivery, Barbara Nickerson is a sallow, thin woman with long, stringy blond hair in need of a wash. Except for a plaid flannel shirt and white athletic socks with red and navy stripes, she is naked from the waist down, a white sheet draped across her lap. Her jeans-wearing husband is sitting beside her, his gray T-shirt emblazoned with PORTLAND. He looks weary, his moustache drooping perhaps even more than usual.

"Kevin, you'd better get that damned crib set up tonight!" says a jumpy, desiccated woman of fifty or so. "Don't you think you've waited long enough?" She paces back and forth the length of the bed, long fingers crisping for a forbidden cigarette.

"Yeah, yeah, yeah," he singsongs to the older woman.

"How you doing, hon?" he asks, turning toward his wife on the bed.

The younger woman flashes him a look of confidential love, of wonderful secrets shared.

"Mom," she says slowly, "why don't you go down to the cafeteria and get yourself something to eat? It's going to be a long night."

"Why should I!" replies her mother, more statement than question.

"Because I told you to," says the daughter. "That's why." She laughs, not unkindly, at her mother.

"Oh, all *right*!" says the grandmother-to-be. "You *guys*! You want I should give Harlan a call and have him go over and help me set up that crib in the morning?"

"Now that'd be real nice, Mom," says Barbara Nickerson. "We'd like that, wouldn't we, Kevin? *Kev-in*?"

Her husband grunts, assenting.

"Yeah, Lurlene, that'd be nice. That'd be real nice."

Down in the Mother-Baby Unit, Hilary Blanchard yawns and blinks several times. The tape deck on the table beside the bed is playing Bach's "Where Sheep May Safely Graze." She's been working for two or three hours, ever since dinner, on her needlepoint, and has almost finished the central figure of the unicorn. Tomorrow morning, after her massage, she'll get started on the fence imprisoning the mythical beast. She'd thought she'd make it into a pillow when it's done. But maybe she should follow her mother's suggestion and have the completed piece stretched onto a canvas, and put it in the baby's room.

Hilary is thirsty, but she knows damned well if she finishes up the bottle of Perrier on the bedside table she'll just have to get up and pee the minute she falls asleep. Oh, well. It's probably totally flat by now, anyway.

Yawning again, Hilary rolls up the needlepoint canvas and puts it into the willow basket on the floor beside her bed.

Back on 4NE, a homely stand-up comedian cracks wise on the TV screen in Room 2. Elizabeth Duncan sighs heavily, dabbing at her glistening nose with the damp and shredded Kleenex. Chief Resident Jan Leigh, her long, dark, shiny hair held back with a tortoiseshell barrette, is attempting to move Elizabeth's baby around, to change the position of its head. Her hand plunged deep within Elizabeth's vagina, she is clearly causing considerable pain, however necessary, to the patient. Despite this, Elizabeth just sighs more heavily, raising her feet, as ordered, their iridescent pink-painted toenails shimmering in the bright light.

In the coffee/supply room, two nurses yawn. One of them pours a cup of coffee for the other.

2242: 10:42 P.M.

Elizabeth Duncan weeps silently, her face contorted.

"*Push,* Elizabeth!" urges Resident Gary Hoffman.

"You're doing fine, Elizabeth! Now *push!*" says Nurse Patti Spooner.

"Push *real hard,* Elizabeth!" says Nursing Student Heather Emmerich, getting into the spirit.

The woman gives a monumental push, her face reddening with the effort.

"Let's give it . . . like two more pushes, Elizabeth!" instructs Dr. Hoffman.

As the patient continues to weep, wiping at her tears with a fresh Kleenex someone has handed her, her husband keeps his eyes on the television screen, where a baby shower is being given for an obnoxious character on Channel 12's *Duet.*

"If you feel like pushing, go ahead and push," says Nurse Patti Spooner. "That's the only way we're going to get this over with!" She strokes Elizabeth's thin blond hair with her hand.

Duet is signing off. Preparations are now made to do a scalp pH test on the baby. Dr. Hoffman puts the cone inside Elizabeth's vagina while the patient weeps, at last making a soft sobbing sound.

As *Star Trek: The Next Generation* comes on, Anesthesiology Resident Robert Goldman enters the room.

211

"I'm going to comfortablize her a little bit," he tells Dr. Hoffman, assuring him that the patient will still be able to push.

Outside, around the nurses' station, the hubbub of shift change is going on. Jaynee, the night unit secretary, has brought a big box of Dunkin' Donuts. Surrounded by doctors and nurses, she opens the box with a dramatic flourish.

"Tah-dah!" she says, laughing. Jelly doughnuts. Chocolate doughnuts. Powdered doughnuts. Glazed doughnuts.

Like a fresh crop discovered by locusts, they are descended upon. Three minutes later, the doughnuts are gone.

CHAPTER FOURTEEN

(Handsome Refugee from Communist Country Finds New Home in Land of the Free.)

CHIEF RESIDENT NICHOLAS ABRUDESCU chews slowly on an oatmeal cookie from the tin somebody brought in this afternoon and sips slowly from his mug of coffee. He thinks about the hydrocephalic baby whose cesarean birth he will probably supervise tonight.

At thirty-five, the tall, handsome Romanian, a reputed ladies' man, is far more qualified than most chiefs. Like other fourth-year residents in obstetrics and gynecology, Nicholas has basic medical schooling, followed by years of residency. With this Eastern European refugee, though, the residency on Pill Hill duplicates training he underwent back in his homeland. Nothing he could do about it, once he came here—arriving with the assurances of American doctors that he knew in Romania, qualified American doctors who told him yes, yes, yes, he'd be a doctor of medicine in this country. What they didn't mention was that he would not be able to practice here without repeating his residency, without additional training.

Nicholas Abrudescu was born in Bucharest in 1953 into a family with distinguished medical credentials. His father, Theodore, is the chief of staff of the nation's general emergency hospital. His mother, Pauline, was the country's first woman associate professor of chemistry; at the time of her death in 1984, she was chief of the department of geology at the university in Bucharest. One aunt is a gynecologist, another aunt and uncle are dentists, a cousin an orthopedic surgeon. His brother Florentin, who is four years younger, followed Nicholas here and is himself doing an OB/GYN residency in Cleveland.

When Nicholas was a young boy, he thought he'd like to be an engineer, but was encouraged to move toward medicine. Going with his father to the hospital, watching him operate, made medicine look exciting. Romania's educational system differs greatly from America's. After the compulsory eight years of elementary school, he went on to high school, where admission is based on strong competition. While the whole school system is free to students, competition for higher education is fierce, and only a few make it. Would-be university students who fail the entrance exams are allowed to retake them two or three times. But ultimate failure means you must do something else. In medicine there's no "pre-med": Future doctors begin preparing right after high school, completing a six-year program, instead of four years after acquiring a bachelor's degree. The first two and a half years of Romanian medical school are pre-med course work—anatomy, physiology, chemistry, and all that.

Dr. Nicholas Abrudescu thinks the American system is superior to Romanian medical training. Here, once you learn something, and pass the course, it's finished. You don't go back over it. So slowly, slowly, you concentrate your mind and energy on a certain area and go deeper and deeper. In Romania you keep wasting your energy for years and years on broad subjects instead of concentrating on one area.

After his six years of medical school in Bucharest, Nicholas passed a very difficult competition to qualify for a three-year residency in obstetrics and gynecology. After that, there were more competitions to determine where he would practice medicine. In Romania, you cannot be a doctor wherever you choose. Hopefully, you get a good position somewhere, and then you lead a good life. You can have either an apartment or a house. You can have up to two houses, a car. Doctors have a higher standard of living than, say, a factory worker. More so than in America. In Romania doctors are at the top, versus here in America, where businessmen and other people are at the top.

After medical school, after completing his residency, Dr. Nicholas Abrudescu developed a secret desire to go to America. Practicing in Bucharest, among his patients were two Romanian women, friends who worked at the American embassy. He delivered a baby for one of them. For the other, he performed an abortion—an operation outlawed for political reasons. This friend, the woman who worked at the American embassy, wanted to help him, to return the favor in some way. It was strange. But all is fate, believes Dr. Nicholas Abrudescu.

He didn't even want to try it, but his girlfriend wanted him, pushed him, to take the ECFMG, the Education Committee of Foreign Medical Graduates, which would waive American medical school requirements. The exam was to be given at the American embassy. And while not exactly forbidden to Romanian physicians by their government, it was regarded as not good for them, not "healthy." Deciding to take the exam, through connections, Nicholas got hold of the *Merck Manual,* a simplified compilation of medical information. It was January 4, and he had three weeks to bone up for the notoriously difficult ECFMG.

On the cold day of the exam, January 26, 1983, the grateful friend who'd received the abortion hid Nicholas Abrudescu in the back of her car, on the floor, whisking him past the Romanian soldiers at the embassy entrance. She pretended to be working overtime, busying herself while he finished the lengthy exam. When all the other exam takers were leaving, she again secreted the doctor in the back of the car, taking him out into the dark night, safely past the soldiers.

In March, Nicholas was surprised to learn that he had passed the exam. He began preparing to leave. Deciding to do so was the most difficult part of all. In 1983 there were two ways to get out of Romania. You could just leave—basically run away. That's nice for the one who leaves, because you just go and never come back. But it's bad for the rest of the family—who suffer and are persecuted. The second way to leave Romania is to ask to leave, which is nice for the rest of the family, if you can call it nice that you are going away for good. At least you're not a fugitive. But for the person who asks permission, it's difficult because it may take years and years to get it.

So Nicholas Abrudescu asked to leave Romania. It took him three years to get official permission. It was nerve-racking, the waiting for permission. If something went wrong, they could have punished him or have had some sort of trial against him. Young people can wait for years; there are people who wait eight, ten years. It's like in Russia, with the Refuseniks. You're allowed to *ask* permission—it's just that you can lose your job, your telephone, your standing in the community, too. Every year there are people who leave, but very few. Finally, Nicholas left, claiming that he was going to America for a fellowship to develop his medical skills, that he would return. He would not return, he knew, and his family knew it, too.

While waiting to go to the United States, he visited other European countries, where he had friends all over. The friends invited him to stay, to practice medicine in France or a number of other countries. Being a refugee from a Communist country, he could have remained anywhere. No, he said, thanking them, he was going to the United States. He liked the sound of the States, of the American system. It was the land of immigrants, so he wanted to get on the boat, to go across the ocean, and to be a doctor here.

Dr. Nicholas Abrudescu expected some surprises, but the biggest surprise of all was discovering that yes, he was a doctor in the United States, but he wouldn't be allowed to practice medicine! It was unbelievable. All over the world, you're either a doctor or you're not. And if you are, you are accorded all the privileges of being a doctor. This is the only country where you must have a license on top of everything else you have. If you go to Canada, this is not true. All over Europe, this is not true—they've never even heard of it! In the United States, the license is your true diploma, and you do not get it until you are fully qualified. That's the American system. That's all. Period. No argument.

He couldn't believe so many people had given him *first-hand* information, these Americans doing their studies in Romania, going back to America every three months, six months, for their vacations. Nicholas had carefully asked them precise questions. And they told him that with his three years of internship and another three years of residency, in America he could go straight to a fellowship.

To get a license to practice medicine in the U.S., you take a test for three days in a row, one minute allotted to answer each question. They take all the medical school, from the beginning to the end. There are two parts, lasting a day and a half each. The first part is all those basic sciences, which are obnoxious. And then the second part is clinical sciences, which are nice until you have to take a *test* on them! Worst of all, they demand that you take both parts at the same time, in a row—at least in Oregon and all the important states. And if you pass one and fail the other, *both* parts are considered failed. And on top of all that, you can take the test only three times!

Nicholas arrived at the worst possible time, when the United States was having a crisis with all the graduates from foreign schools, all these American-born students who couldn't get into medical school here, and then went all over the world, and then came back in waves, expecting to pass themselves off as doctors. This was unheard of in Europe—it was *unbelievable*! And now the Romanian doctor had lost his status as a refugee as far as other countries were concerned. Because he was in the United States, a free country, he couldn't return to Europe—which seemed like a good idea, now that he'd learned of the obstacles ahead. According to the terms of the Geneva Convention, you are considered a "refugee" only as long as you move to a country with a government opposed to the one you are fleeing from.

It was bad. Really, really tough. Nicholas wanted to return to Europe, where he had many friends. Here, he knew nobody. He wasn't sure he'd be able to *take* those exams. Here it was 1983, and he had started medical school in 1972, finishing in 1978. He felt like crying. Biochemistry, anatomy—*aaach*!

In downtown Miami, he slept somewhere disgustingly close to the airport, and lived on three dollars a day. So much noise from the planes taking off and landing! Cockroaches crawling all over him! And Nicholas hates cockroaches, a strange thing because he has no problems with rats or mice or snakes. But cockroaches, something about their shells! He cannot eat lobster for the same reason. He can eat the meat of the lobster, but if you show him the lobster itself, you can take it away.

He had to get away from the planes landing and the cockroaches crunching underfoot. He applied to the American College of Gynecology, and presented his credentials. They had some openings in different places. Openings for residents, people who had just completed the four years of medical school.

Languishing in his roach-ridden room near the Miami airport, Nicholas was offered a position with a hospital in South Africa, and the only reason he turned it down was because South Africa is so much against Communist countries that he could not have been in any sort of contact with his family again.

While he was considering the possibility, getting close to leaving, he was offered a four-year residency in obstetrics and gynecology at Oregon Health Sciences University. He grabbed it and came to Portland. While he'd brought some money with him, it was very tough, living on three bucks a day. Dr. Kirk was so nice to him. He told Nicholas, "Well, if you need money, I can lend it to you, and you can pay me back when you are paid." But Nicholas wouldn't take it, no thank you. He preferred to be on his three bucks a day. But Dr. Kirk was the only one who was nice to him. Looking back now, that makes Nicholas kind of bitter.

Here in Portland, there are nice people in general, but in the residency program, Dr. Kirk and his wife were the only ones who paid any attention to him. The others, they never tried to help him out, never tried to do anything. They didn't even ask him where he was living. They'd just start blushing if he spoke to them. It bugs Nicholas that he thought this was the American system, and then he found out that wasn't true. Before too long, the nicer ones, they would try to be helpful, and wanted to talk. At first, the new resident ended up in a kind of depressing area, in a group of apartments for residents over across the river by Emanuel Hospital. He spent more than a year there, with the Life Flight air ambulance helicopter over his apartment day and night, day and night—Jesus! Really bad.

Now Nicholas has a social life. But then he was alone, he was out of it. His English was okay, mostly because his mother always said it is better to know a foreign language, so he learned English and French. Sure, his English could be improved, but the Romanian accent . . . well, there are times when it is very useful. When an accent such as his is considered attractive, romantic.

Looking back, his second year, 1985, was probably the worst. Second-years work very hard because they're supposed to be in charge of the high-risk OB rotation, which is the most difficult. On top of it, he had to prepare for the FLEX, the licensing examination—because without the license exam, he could never be a doctor in the United States, he could never be a chief resident. Then there was also the *moral* pressure, that you *have* to take and pass this exam. He very seriously started looking into truck driving. He was a good driver. Why not be a truck driver? It is very secure work. Or he could be a guide, like when he was a student back in Bucharest. He could guide groups around the area. Then someone he knew told Nicholas that she and a friend were growing Christmas trees. He could grow Christmas trees. That wouldn't be so bad.

Thinking about it now, it's funny, but at the time, exhausted and worried that he wouldn't pass the FLEX, it was depressing. Every day, he would wake up at five o'clock in the morning, go to the hospital at six, and work until six-thirty P.M. Then he would go downtown to the library and read until ten o'clock, go home around ten-thirty, eat a sandwich, and collapse. Nicholas did this from May until December, and he was ready to *die*. It was the worst, *the* worst. He took the FLEX, and passed it. Then things started improving somewhat. But still there are problems.

The residents are paid very little. Once, they sat around in the coffee/supply room and calculated it. In L&D, if you figure only the hours—not the extra hours, but the hours you're on call and all—after taxes, you get $2.60, $2.70 an hour. It goes up, like $80 a month each year, as you work your way up to being a chief resident. Now it's maybe $2.90, $3.00 an hour! Now he gets something like $1,300, $1,400 a month—that's for being a chief, the highest level! Everybody's paid the same. They just survive. Usually, the husband or the wife, they work, which makes a difference.

All things considered, Nicholas Abrudescu is glad he stayed in the United States. (Not that there was that much choice, once he was here.) He likes this system of medicine better than the one in Romania, where the big hospitals were concentrated, everything state-controlled. The OB/GYN department where Nicholas worked had 450 beds. The whole *hospital* was for obstetrics and gynecology. OHSU doesn't even have thirty beds!

With very few exceptions, the doctors here are well trained. And the nurses, in general, are very good. And—he admits it—the residency program is superior to any he's seen in Europe. *Obviously* superior. The relationships among the staff, residents, and nurses are also very good. The quality of care of sick people is very good, and that's not just because of the doctors, but because of the whole system. In his mind, there's no comparison, really, with the hospitals in Romania.

The availability of good medical care to all people, though, is a real problem in America. It's not a problem in Canada, it's not a problem in Europe, it's not a problem in any other civilized society. He has read that the rate of prematurity is ten times higher here than in Western Europe! And it's well known that the most important factor in preventing prematurity is early prenatal care. It's unbelievable, it's frustrating. They spend an incredible amount of money transplanting organs into people who are incurable, which is nice, but . . . ! They take a four-year-old who is going to die anyway and do experiments transplanting everything, and spend $400,000. Yet no money is spent on preventing prematurity, or on treating simple causes of so many diseases.

But there are so many good things about the system. During his residency, Nicholas has been working all over the city—Good Samaritan, Emanuel, Kaiser, St. Vincent. He did abortions at the Lovejoy Clinic and the Women's Feminist Health Clinic. And there's no place as good as here, nurse-wise. Here, they are the most reliable, the most efficient, the best with the patients. The nurses call you up when they have a problem, compared with other places where they drive you crazy calling you up for nothing—or *not* calling you up for something very serious.

Nicholas was accustomed to working with outstanding people in Romania. His professor of surgery, for example, was the personal doctor to President Nicolae Ceausescu. He was a general surgeon, a member of the French Academy. A big, big shot. And his professor of OB/GYN was the president of the European Society of Obstetrics and Gynecology—and the vice president of the *international* society, here in San Francisco. Two big, important people. Clearly, there are only two people at OHSU who are remarkable in that sense. One is Dr. Kirk. The other is Dr. John Bissonnette.

What makes Paul Kirk remarkable is a mixture. In his case—and Nicholas has thought about him many, many times—he's an extremely intelligent man, a very good clinician. When a situation with a patient is simple, then everybody knows what to do. But when it's complicated, everybody thinks it's one way, and Kirk thinks it's another way, then he's right! In four years Nicholas cannot remember him making *one mistake*. Then, too, Dr. Kirk has a very broad mind. A very good sense of humor. He's very compassionate, very understanding. He can really help you out if you have a problem. Yet he knows how to combine honey with the whip. It's interesting. He knows where to push it—he's very nice, but then can be firm.

The residents aren't afraid of Dr. Kirk. He is respectful of them, and that's why everything works. He makes a big point of emphasizing everybody's dignity. Especially with patients who are sick, so they might feel sort of inferior at that moment. He says you should be more respectful, try to make them feel good, instead of exacerbating what they already have. Like: "You're healthy, they're sick." His wife is marvelous! Nicholas actually told Dr. Kirk one time that they say that at least 50 percent . . . that behind every successful man there is a woman. Nicholas is sure that it's more than 50 percent! Monica Kirk is remarkable, a wonderful person. Oh yeah, she is wonderful, the way she helped him when he first came to Oregon.

You get used to the thirty-six-hour shifts, the sleep deprivation. It's interesting to see that the professors seem to have very unusual resistance to illness. Initially, Nicholas Abrudescu was aiming to do a fellowship. In fact, that's what he thought he was doing when he first arrived, in 1983. But he didn't expect to be doing so many years in a row! He'll see. He'll go into private practice, OB/GYN. And if he feels really frustrated, he'll go back and try to do a fellowship. At least he'll know that's the way to go.

Nothing ever turns out the way you think it will. Nicholas's mother was Jewish, and she tried to raise him in the Jewish religion. But as a product of a Communist society, he doesn't really believe in religion very much. And actually, since his mother died, he doesn't think there is any God. She died a year after Nicholas left, died because he left. Perhaps not 100 percent because of that, but clearly his departure had something to do with it. He knew that his leaving would be tough for her, but this! If he had only known, he would never have left! He returned to Romania for her funeral, and was a little afraid that the authorities would force him to remain, but it didn't happen.

So he must move forward. Nicholas Abrudescu became a U.S. citizen last year. He has decided to accept an offer to practice OB/GYN with a small group of doctors in a small HMO in Quincy, Massachusetts, outside Boston. There was a nice offer from Kaiser, to work with their vast HMO—health maintenance organization—here in Portland. He's worked there a couple of times, knows the people, and has a nice relationship with them. He had some private offers, but if he had decided to remain in Portland, Kaiser would have been his choice. He decided to be closer to his family. Florentin, his brother, is in Cleveland, and it's easier to get to and from Romania from the East Coast, where there are direct flights in both directions.

Not long ago, a friend showed Nicholas something written by a rabbi, something very nice. It said that all that matters in life is what you do with what happens to you, and what you can change in the future. He thinks about that a lot when he remembers... hiding on the floor of the car as he sneaked into the American embassy in Bucharest... brushing off the horrible cockroaches in Miami...being awash in loneliness when first coming to Pill Hill. Nicholas tries to remember all that when the familiar grief floods his soul, when he believes— as he will all his days on this earth—that his beloved mother's heart gave out because he left his homeland.

CHAPTER FIFTEEN

DAY 8: Monday, April 18

("Are you scared, Lisa? Are you scared?" asks the father-to-be, age eighteen.)

1545: 3:45 P.M.

IT'S A BRIGHT BUT overcast day outside the window of the coffee/supply room on Pill Hill's 4NE.

In PAR, in the bed across from one holding a small Vietnamese woman, Elena Martinez is being readied for her scheduled c-section.

In Room 18, Georgia Williams, a robust woman in her mid-thirties, has been examined and is about to go down to the Mother-Baby Unit until the labor with her fifth child has progressed further.

Teenaged Frannie Fenner, who's been trying to lure her tardy child out with promises of *candy! candy!*, is now in Room 8, pushing for all she's worth.

In the Exam Room, awaiting admittance, are a moon-faced black woman and Lisa McDonald, whose chart says she's twenty, but whose childish mannerisms make her seem younger, say fifteen or sixteen. Beside her bed, hopping from one foot to another, is Lisa's boyfriend, Jason, eighteen.

And in Room 2, Marilee Babcock awaits induction for the

birth of her anencephalic baby, an infant with no brain.

As preparations are made to section Mrs. Martinez, the talk is of Elizabeth Duncan, the big, silently weeping blonde from last night. About a half hour after midnight, all that pushing finally resulted in a small baby girl. And at last, they say, the father became animated. In fact, once his daughter was born, he leaped from his chair, kissed his wife, and began dancing around the room, singing a song in Spanish.

As for Elena Martinez, the reason she's getting a cesarean section is that she had one before, a low transverse section in which they had to make a T-incision to make more room to get the baby out. Such an incision necessitates cesarean sections for subsequent births, making it impossible for Mrs. Martinez to have a VBAC—a vaginal birth after cesarean. Sectioning her will also make it easier to perform the tubal ligation she has requested.

The word up from the Mother-Baby Unit is that Darleen Robinson, the "seizure disorder" sectioned on Friday morning, wigged out completely last night. Behaved completely inappropriately with her new baby, then threatened to just take him and leave, they say. The MBU staff had to call the psychiatric department, which sent over someone who suggested she might have a personality disorder secondary to a seizure disorder. Darleen also revealed that she has been abused by her husband. It's a problem, what to do now.

In her room, Hilary Blanchard has heard the screams of Darleen Robinson. How in hell—as she asked a nurse in the room with her at the time—is she supposed to get her rest with that zoo playing outside her door, night and day?

"Is there anything I can get you?" was all the stupid cow of a nurse said in reply.

Sighing heavily, Hilary picks up *The New York Times* Richie brought in earlier. Right there on the front page, Louise Nevelson dead! God, how depressing. She turns to the crossword. One across: *Shadowbox.* That's easy. In neat lettering, one letter per square, the gold Cross pen prints SPAR. Five across: *Dunces.* JERKS? Does that fit with five down, *Designate?* Nope. Oh, well, try ten across: *Asian nanny.* Hilary writes in AMAH. A snap.

Fourteen across: *Kind of duck.* LAME. Fifteen across: *Gal-*

lagher's vaudeville partner. SHEAN. (Eyes suddenly stinging, Hilary remembers her parents singing at a party, while she pretended to be asleep, about a thousand years ago. ("*Absolutely, Mr. Gallagher? Positively, Mr. Shean. . . .*")

In a room across the hall, a woman calls out, loudly: "Nurse! Nurse! I think my waters is broke! Nurse! Nurse?"

1600: 4:00 P.M.

The first incision is made on Mrs. Martinez. Medical student Anina Merrill, delicate and blond behind her mask of soft green paper, is doing small chores, tentatively: cauterizing, holding the pull-back metal retractor.

Eleven minutes after the first incision, an angry-looking little boy is retrieved from Mrs. Martinez's open belly. His color is bluish-red, and his umbilical cord is wrapped—twice!—around his neck. Soon, in the hands of the pediatricians on hand at the side of the operating room, the infant is whomped into a nice rosy pinkness, and wrapped up in warm flannel receiving blankets printed with yellow, blue, and pink ducklings, a blue-and-white-striped knit cap topping his ensemble.

1620: 4:20 P.M.

The staff has been alerted that a woman about to deliver a hydrocephalic baby is being sent over from Emanuel. The baby's brain cortex is half a centimeter, they're told. The infant also has a *meningomyelocele,* a type of neural-tube disorder in which the membrane and spinal cord protrude through a defect in the vertebra. At the very least, the infant will be paraplegic. With such a large head, it will be necessary to section the woman. Furthermore, she is from Laos and speaks very little English.

The woman with the baby with no brain may not be delivering soon. And the word is that the fetus is breech.

"That's good," says Resident Julie Bouchard, nodding her head. "That means the presenting part is firm." This fact of the baby's position will make the birthing easier. If the infant's

227

head, misshapened with no brain, were to lead the way through the birth canal, it could be a messy business.

1711: 5:11 P.M.

Lisa McDonald is settled into Room 2. Her boyfriend, eighteen but acting twelve, is hopping around the delivery room, as though he's eaten a few too many Twinkies this afternoon. He pulls the salmon-colored aluminum miniblinds up: *snaaaap!* Then he sends them back down again: *froooomp!*

Lisa, sallow-faced, with brown eyes and shoulder-length brown hair, scowls at the father of her child. After the third set of *snaaaaps!* and *froooomps!* she speaks.

"Jeez, Jason! Knock it off, will you?"

Lisa's mother sits, smiling, in the rocking chair and shakes her head resignedly. (These kids!)

On Channel 12, a syndicated rerun of *Little House on the Prairie* extolls the joys of family life on the frontier.

In the hall outside, Frannie Fenner's mother sits and talks with a funny and charming young man, the twin brother of Tammy Williams, the recent arrival in Room 4.

Inside Room 4, Resident Brian Clark has ordered Pitocin to induce the labor of thirty-six-and-a-half-weeks-pregnant Tammy. At nineteen, Tammy suffers from HELLP syndrome, an unusual complication of pregnancy. For five days in a row, Tammy had cramps in the middle of her abdomen, and pain in the area of her liver. She didn't know if it was flu or gas pains. Her mother thought it could be hepatitis. With less than a month before her baby was due, Tammy could even have been in labor.

Though she'd been a patient at Pill Hill's clinic all through her pregnancy, someone talked Tammy into going to the emergency room at Providence, across the river, just to make sure there wasn't something really wrong with her. There the doctors quickly figured out that she wasn't in labor. However, they took some blood and ran some tests and found that her platelets—the rodlike things in the blood that cause it to coagulate when something goes wrong—were way down, indi-

228

cating that some pathologic process was going on.

Providence sent her over to The Hill. When she arrived on 4NE, Tammy Williams had no fever, no chills, no nausea, vomiting, or aches. So it wasn't flu. Nor did she have any clear contractions or ruptured membranes. Her cervix was about 50 percent thinned out, about one centimeter dilated; she could have had some contractions already or be on her way effacing, going into labor.

Through this continuing process of elimination, the suspicion developed that Tammy's pregnancy had become toxemic. PIH—pregnancy-induced hypertension, high blood pressure, or toxemia—was the suspect. A blood pressure of 140/90 defines hypertension in pregnancy. When the hypertension is associated with *proteinuria*—protein in the urine—and *edema*—fluid retention in the body tissues—it is defined as *preeclampsia,* the most common form of PIH, and the most worrisome. Its etiology, or cause, is unknown; what is known is how to manage it. If it develops very early in the pregnancy, at twenty-eight weeks or so, the risk to both mother and fetus is all too likely to escalate into severity, and means trouble later on.

What happens, good or bad, to a pregnant woman usually happens to her fetus. The *vasospasm,* the narrowing of vascular channels throughout the body, that accompanies preeclampsia moves throughout the vascular system, and can happen at the placenta. It is thought that a vasospasm can be triggered by changes in the placenta, by an abnormal placenta that is not functioning well. Signals are sent out into the mother's bloodstream, telling her body to increase her blood pressure, that she must take on more body water. In more serious cases, the mother may have seizures. The baby, or the mother, may die. The cure is simple: *Get that baby out of there.*

In the case of Tammy Williams, several classic symptoms of pregnancy-induced hypertension were absent. There was no history of headaches, or of seeing spots. At 130/80, Tammy's blood pressure was elevated, though not enough to make an immediate diagnosis of PIH.

Blood studies were sent off to the lab above the University Hospital's outpatient clinic. Tammy Williams's *hematocrit,* her percentage of red blood cells, was elevated, not going down, as is usual with the increased blood volume that usually accompanies pregnancy. Her blood was concentrated, instead of diluted as it should have been by all the extra fluid. Something was going on in her system, some change in her blood vessels. Fluid that belonged in her blood vessels was escaping into her tissues, causing the edema. Her hematocrit was elevated to 40, much higher than it should be in the third trimester. And Tammy's platelet count was down to 91,000. Normally, it would be between 200,000 and 250,000.

Tammy Williams was officially admitted to 4NE, given a working diagnosis of mild PIH, and started on magnesium sulfate, an ionic solution injected intravenously to raise the seizure threshold level in her brain. Her dates—the time of her last menstrual period—were looked at, her cervix was examined, and it was confirmed that she was truly thirty-six-and-a-half-weeks along. At this late stage, the chances of Tammy's baby having lung disease, the great worry with preemies, was low. The decision was made to "pit" the nineteen-year-old, to induce labor with a Pitocin drip.

Pitocin is the synthetic form of *oxytocin,* the uterine contraction-stimulating hormone released by the brain's pituitary gland when a woman goes into labor. Once the woman is delivered, the baby's sucking and other nipple stimulation releases more oxytocin from the brain, causing the muscles around the sacs in the breast to contract, aiding the expression of milk.

Commonly, Pitocin is used for two purposes. The first—as in the case of Tammy Williams—is to put a woman into labor. If her cervix isn't favorable, and it's not possible to start labor by rupturing her membranes, she may receive Pitocin. Once she's been started on the synthetic hormone, over a period of minutes or hours, her contractions will then pick up.

The second use for Pitocin is to aid a woman whose labor has already begun, but isn't going well. There may be a number of reasons for a dysfunctional labor pattern. The woman may, for example, have an anomalous uterus, be a *"grand multip"* who has undergone many deliveries, or simply have an extremely large baby inside her. Whatever the cause, the result can be a uterus that isn't efficient, whose muscles are not contracting in the necessary, coordinated fashion—from the top of the uterus down so that the baby is pushed out. Instead, the uterus just spasms, much like a heart undergoing coronary arrest. In these cases, Pitocin is used to augment labor, to start more effective labor patterns.

Generally, an "effective labor pattern" is defined as approximately three good and regular contractions within a ten-minute period. There are various ways to measure the effectiveness of a woman's contractions, one of which is putting an interuterine pressure catheter inside the uterus, measuring the quantity or strength of these contractions. What it comes down to is this: If a woman has a labor that doesn't seem to be progressing, the doctors can monitor her contractions and their strength. And if the contractions don't seem to represent a normal, adequate pattern, she may be given Pitocin to move things along.

For Tammy, as the hours slowly progressed, what started out looking like garden-variety PIH came to resemble something far more serious. Tammy Williams had HELLP syndrome, a dangerous variation of pregnancy-induced hypertension. In this awkward acronym, H = hemolysis, for the destruction of the red blood cells in the peripheral vasculature; EL = elevated liver enzymes, in Tammy's case up from the normal 50 to 101; LP = low platelets. In general, pregnancies that are, in medspeak, "complicated" by preeclampsia and HELLP syndrome have "poor maternal and perinatal outcome." Up to 60 percent of the babies die; up to 25 percent of the mothers can die.

The two interests, that of mother and unborn child, must be balanced in getting the baby delivered. Is the pregnancy far enough advanced that the child will survive after delivery, with lungs mature enough to live? If not, can you buy some time by ordering complete hospital bed rest? Is the cervix "favorable," or is a cesarean section necessary? Dilly-dally too long, and the condition can progress suddenly. The mother can go into seizure. Such women need close monitoring, usually in the hospital. Decisions about delivery are made day by day, hour by hour.

During her long, Pitocin-induced labor, Tammy's platelets dropped even further, from 91,000 at admission all the way down to 61,000, dangerously below the normal platelet count of 200,000 to 250,000. The only cure—already set into motion—is to get the placenta and the baby out of the teenager. Then, whatever caused this case of HELLP syndrome will go away, and Tammy will get better on her own.

Nobody except Tammy knows who the father of her baby is. Nobody cares. What matters is that *both* Tammy and the infant come through this okay. Both of them.

1805: 6:05 P.M.

The troops are gathered around the nurses' station for Board Rounds, to run down the full house. Dr. Amanda Clark is the staff doctor.

Tammy Williams, the HELLP syndrome patient in Room 4, is being monitored very carefully.

Fern Sampson, in Room 10, is alcoholic and says that if we don't give her something for the pain, she'll start drinking again.

Marilee Babcock, being induced for her anancephalic baby, has had no prenatal care whatever. She says she doesn't want to either see or hold her baby after it is born. Her first baby died of SIDS, and she has one living child. There are a number of friends with her in Room 2, and the nurses have reason to believe she's shooting up with them, even as she labors.

"They're really little and simple," Resident Tracey Delaplain says of Lisa McDonald and her boyfriend in Room 2. "The dad says he's eighteen. You'll think he's thirteen and a half. She says she's twenty. Fifteen or sixteen come to mind."

Joni Phillips, the asthmatic who wanted her tubes tied after the birth, "says she doesn't do IV drugs, but she does do cocaine," reports Med Student Anina Merrill. And the cocaine screen on the baby showed positive.

Muong Phanh, the Laotian woman who'll be sectioned for her hydrocephalic baby, has arrived and will soon be tucked in here.

Board Rounds completed, Dr. Amanda Clark announces

232

that she's going home to cut the grass, and will come back. Walking to the elevator, Dr. Clark passes Fili Cox, who is pushing the wheeled mop bucket from the Special Delivery Room at the end of the hall.

1948: 7:48 P.M.

Cammie Edwards and her tired, sad-faced mother have arrived to take baby Timothy home. Earlier, the INCU nurses bickered about who would have the privilege of feeding the tiny red-haired preemie his last bottle. But Timothy's grandmother and wispy mother don't have the proper court papers to pick him up, and they leave empty-handed.

They'll be back tomorrow morning, Cammie's mother wearily assures the nurses. Mother and grandmother walk slowly down the hall to the elevator, the older woman gently cupping the elbow of the younger one, preventing her from weaving her unsteady way into a chair or a gurney or a wall. The only sound is the *clop-clop-clop* of the young drug addict's sandals on the freshly mopped floor.

2010: 8:10 P.M.

Frannie Fenner's mother, herself not yet forty, staggers out of her teenaged daughter's room, weeping. She is exhausted. A nurse, noticing, gets her a glass of Sprite and leads her down to the Family Waiting Room. She'll come and fetch her when there's been some change.

"Promise?" asks Frannie's mother.

"Scout's honor," replies the nurse, grinning.

In Room 2, Lisa McDonald is weeping, and tells Resident Brian Clark she wants something for the pain. He tells her he'll arrange for some Demerol.

At the foot of the bed, Jason, the curly-haired father-to-be, hops around, squirming with excitement.

"Are you *scared*, Lisa?" he asks. "Are you *scared?*"

On the television screen above, the furry alien called Alf

233

enters the young girl named Lynn in a beauty contest.

"I want some cookies or something," Jason whines. "Why wouldn't you let us stop at the Seven-Eleven for some Ho Ho's or some Twinkies or something before we came here? Your mom would've stopped if you'd of let her. You are *so selfish,* Lisa!"

"Yeah, right, Jason! I'm the selfish one 'cause I don't want to have a baby right there in the backseat of my mom's car! You are nothing but a little pig, you brat," says his laboring girlfriend.

"Well, we *started* the baby in the backseat of that car," says the sugar junkie, briefly chastened. "So are we supposed to get married or what? You never did say."

"Jeez," says Lisa. "I don't want to talk about this *now*! Why don't you go find a candy machine or something and leave me alone?"

2030: 8:30 P.M.

Muong Phanh, the Laotian woman, is lying in Room 8, the fetal monitor strap across her belly. She's been in the United States since 1980, and her American husband's current residence is the Oregon State Correctional Institution in Salem, some forty miles to the south.

It was only when an ultrasound was done today that her baby's condition was known. Had there been more prenatal care, including a fairly routine alpha-feto protein test, the meningomyelocele and hydrocephalus might have been detected. Then, at least, there would have been an option to terminate the pregnancy in its earlier stages.

Muong wants to know if the cesarean section will take place today or tomorrow. Resident Brian Clark doesn't know. She wants to know when she should have her people come. Dr. Clark tells her to have them plan to be here all day. And that she'll be going down to the Mother-Baby Unit for now.

In odd, halting English, Muong tells the resident that she wants to have her tubes tied. This will be her fourth child and that is enough, she insists.

"No more baby!" says the Laotian woman. "No more baby! Plenty baby now!"

2101: 9:01 P.M.

Dr. Amanda Clark is back, half of her grass cut.

"It's never been that tall," she tells Fili, who carries a stack of flannel baby blankets from the coffee/supply room shelves. "The mower kept quitting. It makes me wonder why I fertilized it a couple of weeks ago!"

2105: 9:05 P.M.

Down in the Mother-Baby Unit, a drama unfolds. The cast includes five nurses and the nursing supervisor, two security guards (one male, one female), and a pediatrician. Darleen Robinson, her husband, and their newborn son are ready to make their escape from Pill Hill.

Darleen had been lying, having what she calls "flighty thoughts," and telling the staff that she didn't know where she and her husband were going to stay. While she has been officially discharged from the hospital, there is a court hold on the baby. The hospital social worker and the psychiatric department are involved now. Darleen and her husband returned just to take their baby son.

Thwarted, they become violent.

"You can't take my baby!" howls Darleen.

"I've got to get out of this hospital!" bellows her husband. "I've got to go home and blow up at something before I really hurt someone!"

He leaves, barreling down the hall and through the swinging doors.

"I'm glad the fucker went home!" Darleen announces, in a swift, shrill shift of loyalties.

A half hour later, when a nurse asks, "How're you doing?" Darleen beams.

"I'm just *wonderful!*" she replies in evident sincerity.

An MBU nurse calls up from the third floor to L&D.

"This is Holly," she says. "I'm with Liz Brownell, and she's in labor, and she's dilated to six, and she keeps saying, 'Please don't leave me, don't go!' So I'm going to stay with her. I'll come up with her."

Outside the window of the coffee/supply room, rain has made everything shiny: The leaves on the blooming rhododendron bushes in the parking lot, the oldish, banged-up cars of the residents lucky enough to be assigned parking places, the trash cans and dumpsters, the cement surfaces.

Filipinas Mugas Cox restocks the Jiffy cart with supplies. Betadine and little flannel blankets printed with cartoonlike baby animals join the other equipment that will be used in caring for the mothers and their babies born tonight.

In Room 4, Tammy Williams's contractions are closer together, and harder. The eighteen-year-old with HELLP syndrome clings hard to the hand of her twin brother, who grimaces empathically, reflecting each of Tammy's pains.

"It's okay, Tam," he says. "It's all going to be okay."

Down the hall from the Family Waiting Room come Frannie Fenner's husband and mother, the latter looking much improved.

Resident Brian Clark examines Muong Phanh, still modestly wearing panties beneath her hospital gown. A decision is made to section the Laotian woman tonight.

"Do we have to start thinking about diverting people to other hospitals?" Nurse Molly Wilson asks Dr. Amanda Clark.

"Yes, that's what I'm trying to do—as soon as I can get a *phone*," replies Mandy Clark.

Plans are made for Muong Phanh's section. Neurosurgery has been alerted, in case something can be done for the hydrocephalic baby coming up. At the same time, a close eye is being kept on Room 4's Tammy Williams, whose baby's heart tones are down. She, too, may need to be sectioned tonight.

"We're too busy, as usual, and I'm calling to see if you're up for a few hits," says Dr. Amanda Clark, on the phone to Good Samaritan Hospital in Northwest Portland.

2220: 10:20 P.M.

Preparations continue for Muong Phanh's section. Neurosurgery isn't here, but they say they probably wouldn't do surgery on the baby until morning, anyway.

Frannie Fenner gets an epidural.

In the hallway outside her room, Resident Brian Clark talks with Anesthesiology Resident Tom Emmons about Frannie.

"Well, what do you think? We got a section here?"

"Naw," drawls Dr. Emmons. "They say we're going to slam on her for about another hour. See what the Pitocin does."

2244: 10:44 P.M.

The Doctors Clark, Mandy and Brian, are in the scrub room with Chief Resident Nicholas Abrudescu, trying to decide how to handle Muong Phanh's request for a tubal ligation. Her poor English places them in a quandary. She seems to understand that her baby will either die or be grossly handicapped. But you never know. And, too, she does have three other children at home. They decide to honor her request, performing the tubal in OR2, right after the cesarean section.

A few minutes later, with Dr. Abrudescu across the operating table and Staff Doctor Amanda Clark behind him, Resident Brian Clark makes the low transverse cut in the tiny Laotian woman's huge belly. Using a large square of gauze, a medical student standing beside Dr. Abrudescu sponges blood from the smile-shaped cut, revealing the subcutaneous fatty layer.

Dr. Brian Clark scalpels deftly through this layer into the fascia. Scissors are used to cut and extend the fascial layer. Again, scissors are used to release fascia and muscles from the anterior abdominal wall, creating a wound opening large

237

enough to accept the delivery of a baby—in this case an infant with an enormous head. The muscles are then separated, revealing the glistening thin peritoneal lining of the abdominal cavity.

Using tweezer-shaped forceps, Brian Clark pulls up the peritoneal layer covering Muong's internal organs and opens it with scissors. The Richardson retractor holds back the wrapping tissues, the many-layered opening, revealing the gravid uterus with its malformed child.

The only sound in OR2 is the slurp of the device that cleans up excess blood.

Again using the scalpel, Brian Clark cuts the outer layers of the uterus. The glistening blue amniotic sac with its unfortunate baby is revealed. The fetal head position is quickly checked. Two fingers are inserted into the womb, between the uterine muscle and the thin amniotic sac. Using bandage scissors, the wound is enlarged from side to side.

Gently, with an Allis clamp, the bag of waters is stabbed and broken. The fluids gush bloodily from the woman's belly.

Finally, Dr. Brian Clark reaches into the crimson wound, bringing into the world the muskmelon-sized head of a small baby girl with lovely oriental features. The reverent, heavy silence continues over the *slurp!* of the blood-sucking machine, and the umbilical cord is clamped, then severed.

Five minutes have passed since the first cut was made. As expected, there is a meningomyelocele in the baby's back, an opening in her spine.

Finally, someone speaks.

"Poor little peanut," says a nurse softly.

CHAPTER SIXTEEN

DAY 9: Tuesday, April 19

("You guys need improvement!"
scrawls the spastic patient, gazing at
the resident's crotch.)

1536: 3:36 P.M.

A STARTING-TO-RAIN TUESDAY AFTERNOON, with half of 4NE's labor and delivery rooms empty.

In PAR, Anita Johnson, who came in at 1:10 A.M. and had a standard vaginal delivery of a son less than two hours later, is recovering from her tubal ligation.

In Room 16, Alicia Delgado is in the early stages of labor and is about to be shipped back down to the Mother-Baby Unit until she makes more progress.

In the Exam Room are Melissa Westheimer and Deneesha Merritt, going through admission procedures. (At least, that's what they hope.)

And in Room 10, Tammy Williams, the eighteen-year-old with HELLP syndrome, continues her difficult labor. Tammy's now-somber twin brother sits in a chair alongside the bed, holding her pale, damp hand, stroking it with his two strong ones. In soft soliloquy, he speaks now of a summer day when they were eight years old and ventured forth into the world, foraging for soda-pop bottles to cash in. Her eyes shut, his

239

sister smiles weakly, nodding from time to time. Curled up like a small child, their exhausted mother dozes in an armchair on the other side of the bed, delicately snoring under a white thermal blanket.

Down in the Mother-Baby Unit, new parents Lisa McDonald and her giddy boyfriend, Jason, admire their new son, Jovian, born at 2:30 this morning, weighing five and a half pounds. Lisa was in hard labor for forty-five minutes, and Jovian was delivered by a nurse-midwife. ("Some small lady with short hair," recalls Jason, holding his little son, bouncing the sleeping newborn until he awakens, squalling.)

"Oh, God, Jason," says Lisa in exasperation, "will you put that kid *down?*"

Two doors down in the MBU, Frannie Fenner and her family admire Jacob, who was finally born at 2:35 A.M., five minutes after Lisa and Jason's little boy. Eighteen-year-old Frannie is drained, still weary from her difficult eight-hour labor induced last evening. A few of the toys offered the baby are arranged in the bassinet: a small teddy bear made of real fur, a tiny Raggedy Andy doll, and a silver rattle.

The baby, who weighs nine pounds and ten ounces, sleeps soundly after his long and arduous journey. His lips are curved upward.

"I think he's smiling, Frannie," announces the new grandmother. "I don't care *what* they say—I know the difference between a smile and gas!" The baby sleeps on.

"He has a big head," says the young woman in the bed. "It was a long, hard push! I feel one hundred percent better!"

"Is that *all,* Frannie?" asks her mother, laughing. The older woman is considerably cheerier, having finally gotten six straight hours of sleep.

"When that baby came out, I was just exhausted!" says the new grandmother. She flew up from her Southern California home Sunday night, when Frannie called and told her the time was at hand.

"This is the first boy in our family for thirty-five years—on my husband's side, and on my side, too," she tells a nurse

240

in the room. "So we're *double* proud!" She smiles at her young blond daughter, leaning down to give her a big hug.

Next door to Frannie Fenner's room, Pearl Monley, the young black woman whose second child was born Sunday, talks with her boyfriend, Clarence, about how different it is now from seven years ago, when their daughter Renaya was born here.

"Remember how they wouldn't let both you and my sister Ruth in the labor room with me at the same time?"

The boyfriend, still wearing a knit cap covering most of his graying hair, nods.

"And now they make you have the baby in the room here with you afterwards. Whether you like it or not."

Another silent nod.

"I mean, it's okay, 'cause he's such a good baby. But some of us would just as soon rest up after having a baby."

Again, there's no spoken reply.

"You know what I mean, Clarence? Clarence, are you even *listening* to me?"

"Yeah, baby, I'm listening to you," comes the reply, gruff and baritone. "You're not the only one who's tired around here, you know."

Four floors down, Marilee Babcock's baby, brainless and unnamed, lies cold and still. Edgar Allan Poe could have designed the morgue in the basement of North Hospital. Tucked into the bowels of the building, the morgue is reached by going down a darkened subterranean hall with water pipes dripping overhead. The room is small and very cold, its white paint peeling, curling away from chill, damp walls.

On a metal shelf lies the small bundle tagged BABY BAB-COCK. The dead infant is snugly wrapped in a flannel receiving blanket printed with brightly hued baby animals. A pink-and-white-striped knit cap covers her lifeless head, hides the steep slope at the back where a brain should be. Except for the sloping head, Marilee Babcock's dead baby just looks like any FLK, Funny-Looking Kid, her lips kind of bulgy, something odd about the ears, maybe.

On the shelf opposite BABY BABCOCK rests a lumpy white plastic bag, filled with God only knows what.

1740: 5:40 P.M.

Time for Board Rounds.

The cast during this summary of patients both in L&D and the Mother-Baby Unit varies. This afternoon, fifteen people crowd around the nurses' station: one staff doctor, Amanda Clark, and two chief residents—Liz Newhall and Nicholas Abrudescu; Anesthesiology Resident Amy Ream; OB/GYN Residents Linda Moore, Karen Hill, Gary Hoffman, and Paul Brenc (Family Practice Resident Brenc, as of eight this morning, made the scheduled switch in rotations. This morning, he was a pediatrician, now he is an obstetrician); Medical Students Andy Su, Anina Merrill, and Terry Johnson; Nurses Marjorie Wizenreid and Julie Rosen; Nurse-Midwife Linda Lutz; Unit Secretary Diane Kuriatnyk.

1819: 6:18 P.M.

From the eleventh-floor skybridge between North and South hospitals, the panorama—usually dramatic—is even more gorgeous than usual. Holding large plastic bags filled with white thermal blankets, a brisk young man in white jacket is momentarily stilled as he gazes north and east at the Cascade Mountain range displayed in sharp, vivid relief against a sky arrayed in shades of blue and gray. There's just a suggestion of the pink that comes before sunset. The huge Japanese cherry tree below the bridge has shed its pale pink blooms, and birds chirp noisily on the nearby roof, contrasting with the huge, silent, ever-present construction machines.

From North Hospital trot three young women, nurses from 4NE's Intermediate Neonatal Care Unit, on their way across the skybridge to South Hospital's third-floor cafeteria. With a cheerful spring to their steps, they are laughing about something one of them overheard a young mother saying to her newborn.

" 'So what's it gonna be, kid? Law or medicine? Make up your mind!' That's what she said, honest!"

In the cafeteria, Chief Resident Elizabeth Newhall goes through the cafeteria line, shepherding her three children: Kate, nine, Joseph, six, and one-year-old Sam. It's slow back in L&D, giving her a rare moment to play mother.

Dr. Newhall is famed among the residents for a number of singular attributes. There is, of course, her beauty—the tall, slim figure, the strong-featured face with its stunning smile. Then there's her pleasant nature, her sense of humor with the hearty, unself-conscious laugh. Above all, what elicits the most admiration (and downright mystification) is Liz Newhall's ability to get by with almost no sleep. Throughout the four years of her residency, which included the birth of young Sam a year ago, she has seldom complained about anything.

Right now, what the chief resident is doing is making sure that all three of her kids eat at least some dinner before they start on the ice cream. Perhaps because she isn't preoccupied by some patient at the moment, she notices the sound of the Life Flight helicopter outside, probably bringing some car accident victim up Pill Hill. Maybe saving a life, maybe not. And as she half-listens to the chopper, as she points to her son Joe's french fries, Liz Newhall thinks of the original Joe.

There's something Liz thinks of as the "pilot gene." Her father certainly had it. And her older brother Joe, first son of his father's first wife, a woman who died in her twenties, had it too. Joe went to the Air Force Academy at seventeen, became a pilot like his father, and was killed in Vietnam in 1968. He was one of the lost ones, her half brother, the ones you never really found out about. An elite pilot from the Air Force Academy, Joe was part of a squadron whose job it was to rescue downed pilots. And they saw his plane crash. But maybe he bailed out first, into Laos.

Officially, Joe was listed as "missing in action." Hell for his family, for his father and sisters and brothers. And for his wife, who'd dropped out of college to marry him, and their two little kids. Liz was sixteen, a high school sophomore, when Joe died.

They never had a funeral for Joe, Liz thinks now. Not

even some kind of memorial service. One of these days, they've got to do that.

It's been a long, tough slog for Liz since she began medical school at the University of California at Davis in 1975, thirteen long years ago. Most of those she started with have long since finished their residencies, are well into their careers. Mark Nichols, director of the OB/GYN residency program here, was a med-school classmate. So was Liz Newhall's own husband, Jim. But she had three kids, and had to jump through a few other hoops before she found what she really wanted to do.

Elizabeth Pirruccello—spelled like Mississippi, Jim says, only with different letters—was born into an interesting family. Father, son of Italian immigrants, was trained as a lawyer, but ended up instead as an Air Force pilot. Mother, daughter of Swedish immigrants, married the widowed Colonel Pirruccello, and took on his two young sons, as well as producing three more children: Elizabeth was the middle child of the second set.

The family moved around a lot. Topeka, Kansas, where Liz was born. Dayton, Ohio. Rhode Island. Alabama; Paris, France. Back to Ohio, then to Lompoc, California. When Liz was in the eighth grade, her father retired to San Francisco. There she was, this nice Catholic girl in a military family, dropped right smack into 1966 San Francisco. Made her kind of schizophrenic for the rest of her life, Liz figures. Maybe that's why she's a Deadhead, a diehard fan of The Grateful Dead. Though med school, residency, and three kids kind of put a crimp in that.

Liz remembers the very moment she decided to become a doctor. She was driving around San Francisco with her father and older sister, Mary, the latter getting ready to go to college. They were discussing what Mary could be when she grew up. A lawyer? A teacher? A doctor? Sitting in the backseat of her father's car, Liz Pirruccello decided then and there. *A doctor! That's a really good idea! That's what I'll do!*

Financing it would be tricky, but possible. Luck sometimes arrives in grisly guise. When Liz was seventeen, she had an accident on a sailboat that resulted in a little educational nest egg. What the teenaged Liz meant to do was to push a friend into the water. Instead, she walked through a just-cleaned plate-glass window, sat down on it, and spent the next few weeks in the hospital. Those were the days before big lawsuits, and the boat's owners bought her off for $11,000, which really came in handy when it came time for medical school. She had a Regents' scholarship. Then there were the loans that everybody ends up taking out. Which will hopefully be paid off sometime before menopause.

She survived San Francisco's Lowell High School. A very academic school that was, in the late sixties, very radical, with even the teachers organizing demonstrations. She was very proper, very straight, very repressed. Then when she started freshman year at UC Davis, it was *vroooom!* I'll try this... I'll try that... I'll try that.... She skied her brains out, and got her pre-med requirements done clandestinely, majoring in biochemistry without ever being so uncool as to let on that, all along, the plan was medical school.

Liz had a choice of staying on at Davis for med school, or going to Columbia University. But it was nutty to get into so much debt, to be that far away, just for the adventure of living in New York.

Liz Pirruccello and Jim Newhall met during their first year of med school. Both were with other partners, and she was still in her wild and rowdy stage, and they didn't get around to falling in love until their second year. Liz agreed to marry him during their third year, as long as he didn't cut his luxuriant tresses shorter than shoulder length for the ceremony.

The couple promptly had Kate, which produced panic. Don't worry, said Jim Newhall, I'm not really having a great time. I'll just drop down to half-time, take care of the baby while you finish up.

That was the way their marriage would progress: one mate going full-bore while the other held down the fort at home. The family moved to Spokane, where Liz started an internship in internal medicine.

Internal medicine was the shits. Nothing but old dying people. Very depressing. While Jim did his residency, Liz worked in emergency medicine. Joe—named after her missing brother—was born in 1981, and Liz often toted the infant and a baby-sitter to the Spokane emergency room when she had a twenty-four-hour shift.

All along, though, she had this yearning for something more personal, more connected to people. Even before she went to medical school, Liz had been interested in women's health care, giving abortion and birth-control advice, and working in a free clinic in Davis. All through med school, for fun, she did women's health work at the free clinic a couple of nights a week. But that was fun, and work wasn't supposed to be fun. She was supposed to be the best of the best, the smartest of the smartest. And if you were really smart, you were an internist.

To be honest, going from that ill-fated year as an internal medicine resident to emergency medicine was mainly because it was easy, it paid well, and Liz could take care of her children. Having two young kids at home, working only one day a week made her about as nuts as she'd ever been.

So when Jim finished his residency, it was *no decision*. Obviously, Liz had to go into obstetrics and gynecology. It was clear to the Newhalls that it was important to do work that you love. More important than doing work that pays well. More important than doing work stamped CERTIFIED INTELLECTUAL by the American Medical Association.

Liz Newhall's next step was to get into an OB/GYN residency program, either in Seattle or back to UC Davis. However, since Portland was in between the two cities, and their old med-school crony Mark Nichols was running Pill Hill's residency program, it seemed only prudent to drop by and say hello.

It turned out there were other friends here. And then one day Liz drove over the bridge to Sauvie Island. Simply looking for an affordable place with some acreage, she found a generous chunk of land with the island's original game warden's cabin. Though in crummy shape, the house was fixable and plunked down right in the middle of an Eden-like setting. Jim, a burgeoning gardener, fell in love with it, too. They bought the house immediately. It is the perfect place to raise children, to have a horse, to grow flowers and vegetables, to cultivate a fruit orchard.

Liz wanted OHSU, and the school wanted her as a resident. All along, it's been a happy match. She was so happy to do something she liked, finally to find her niche in medicine. She'd been out on her own for five years, and the stresses were certainly there. But she loves the work—is probably the happiest resident on The Hill, commuting from her island Eden.

The day Liz Newhall started delivering babies, she knew she was a goner. She probably cried the first one hundred babies she delivered. Right away, she knew she wasn't going to get through this residency without having one more child of her own. So she made a deal with Jim: She'd agree to live on Sauvie Island forever if he'd agree to father one more child. That's how Sam happened, a little red-haired boy born a year ago, last April.

The sleep deprivation hasn't even gotten to her. She never really needed a lot of sleep. You can get up in the middle of the night and not ever feel grouchy, because once you're there, you get so totally into it. Time is completely irrelevant. It's just such a privilege to become a part of such a wonderful time in people's lives. Not that it always is at the university. Sometimes, you hand mothers their babies, and they say, "I don't want it! Clean it up! Get it away from me!" But by and large, hopefully, it's a happy experience.

Labor and Delivery here—anywhere—is such an intense little microcosm. The way Liz Newhall sees it, until our society deals with many of the ills that present themselves on 4NE— the violence, drug addiction, alcoholism, abuse of women, reproductive rights being threatened, and all the rest—they're just going to keep being contributed to. What the doctors and nurses up here have to deal with is completely outside their range to affect.

You're just constantly in a state of reaction to what's happening. And it's really mild here. Take a look: Go to Los Angeles, go to New York. It's really important for people to be aware of the reality of the huddled masses.

One-year-old Sam Newhall, who has his mother's coppery red hair, drops his cookie on the floor of South Hospital's cafeteria. He begins to wail unconsolably.

Hilary Blanchard lies atop her bed, momentarily content after her catered dinner. Tonight, it was salmon in a dill sauce, tiny cheese rounds, shredded red cabbage, and cold fresh asparagus, set off by sprigs of lilac and arranged beautifully on a bamboo tray. And all for just $8.00 per tray, marvels her mother, whose dinner also arrived from Briggs & Crampton. The grandmother-to-be is back to her knitting, the needles clicking in counterpoint to the desultory conversation. Lying back on the pillow, Hilary is trying to decide if she should put in a little more time on the needlepoint. If she spends another hour or so, she'll be able to finish the central unicorn figure. Even the horn.

A vase of orchids reposes on a table, which also holds a photograph of a horse in a silver frame. The sound is muted on the forgotten television set above, on which various celebrities are pigeonholed, silently moving their mouths in a game of *Jeopardy!* Hilary leans over the side of her bed to pick up her needlepoint from the willow basket.

Hilary Blanchard isn't the only long-term MBU resident who finds the hospital food distasteful. At the moment, twenty-two-year-old Debbie Pellegrini slumps in her wheelchair by the nurses' station and drools, but not over the evening's repast. A stroke several years ago left an intelligent, still-alert Debbie palsied and wheelchair-bound. While the stroke physically disfigured her, it did nothing to quench her vigorous sexual yearnings. Her parents and siblings gave up on her three or four years ago.

Since then, the young woman has lived alone, surviving on public assistance, which includes regular visits from a caseworker. But something has to be done, according to the last caseworker report. Debbie leaves unfinished food around her dark, malodorous apartment, ankle-deep in rodent feces, papers, and dirty clothing.

And then there's the matter of the pregnancy. The child's father is thought to be Debbie's landlord, but given her caseworker-documented custom of sitting on the front porch pantyless, her skirt hiked up above her waist, paternity remains, as they say, ambiguous.

Debbie's weeks-long residence in MBU is plainly due to the fact that nobody knows what to do with her, where to put her. The young woman is alone in her staunch belief that she'll be able to tend to her baby independently. The current plan is to find a foster home willing to care for both Debbie and her newborn.

In the meantime, Debbie Pellegrini lives directly across the hall from Hilary Blanchard, on the third floor of North Hospital atop Pill Hill, in the Mother-Baby Unit where her sheer cleverness and sense of humor are the source of both amusement and consternation to the staff. More than once, she has conned someone into phoning out for Domino's Pizza, triumphantly sharing her booty with the nurses and residents. And she has the hots for DDH, her yen for the handsome resident Gary Hoffman less hidden than similar feelings among MBU's more physically fit occupants and staff.

This evening, though, Debbie has confined her attentions to making drooly sounds addressed to DDH. Unable to make herself understood verbally, she gets a piece of paper and a ballpoint and scrawls out a message to the object of her affections: YOU GUYS NEED IMPROVEMENT!

The resident laughs in agreement.

"We sure do, Debbie!" says Gary Hoffman, pausing to give her arm a pat before continuing on his round of patients. "We sure do!"

2129: 9:29 P.M.

Linda Lieber, in to have her third baby, is settled into Room 10.

In Room 8, Betsy Steen's husband is convinced someone has given his wife something to make her sleepy. He won't believe she hasn't been given any medication, nothing at all.

"Harold," says Betsy, whose long blond hair is in braids, "I told you nobody gave me anything. Now will you put a sock in it?"

"I want to know what's going on!" he fumes furiously. Standing next to him, another man, huge, tells Nurse Patti Spooner that he's Betsy's "guardian angel."

"You're some kind of angel, I'm Mother Teresa," retorts the laboring woman. She turns her head toward the nurse. "Meet my big brother Chester. Thinks he's looking out for me. Can't seem to get out of the habit. Gets a little excited every so often."

"And I'm missing *Moonlighting*!" brother Chester adds, his face beginning to redden.

Everyone laughs, the tension broken.

"How do you work the TV?" asks Betsy. "Chester doesn't get his weekly hit of Cybill Shepherd, he gets downright dangerous!"

Nurse Patti Spooner happily obliges, deftly demonstrating how the remote control works. With a snap of the device, the group sees Bruce Willis and Cybill Shepherd materialize on the screen above, Maddie and Addison squaring off in a limp satire of Shakespeare's *The Taming of the Shrew*.

"All *riiiiight*!" says brother Chester, Betsy Steen's guardian angel. "That's more *like* it!" He settles his ample rump into an armchair.

Nurse Patti Spooner exits Room 8.

"Chester, you weren't such an ox, I'd jump right out of this bed and clobber you upside the head," says Betsy Steen, who indeed *is* sleepy. "You both stop scaring the nurses right this minute or I'm sending you home, hear?"

CHAPTER SEVENTEEN

DAY 10: Wednesday, April 20

("I wanna go! I wanna go!" shrieks the three-year-old at the sight of his emerging sister.)

1521: 3:21 P.M.

HAVING ARRIVED AT MIDNIGHT and labored all through the night and day, a plump oriental woman named Melissa Sugawa finally produces a girl. Born face first, the poor baby looks like a boxer after a particularly bad bout, everyone agrees.

Down in the MBU, a blond male nurse named Tom bottle-feeds little Jovian, son of the childlike Lisa McDonald and her boyfriend, Jason. Passing by their room, he was repeatedly struck by how the young parents seemed to be playing with the newborn as though he were a doll, almost taunting him. Finally, the nurse decided to feed the hapless infant himself.

In the room directly across the hall, Muong Phanh recovers from last night's cesarean section and talks with two other Laotian women. Why, they ask her, why? Why did she let the doctors do something to her so that she can never have another baby? Muong weeps, insisting that nobody told her there would be something wrong with this new baby.

On the twelfth floor of South Hospital, in the part known

251

as Doernbecher Children's Hospital, Muong's daughter Jennifer lies listlessly in her crib, a portion of the excess fluid removed from her brain. While her head is still huge, it is grotesque only in relation to her small body. Jennifer is beautiful, the oriental cast of her features lending a piquancy, an ineffable loveliness to her face.

A nurse approaches the bed with a bottle, preparing to pick up and feed Muong's baby.

"Hello, sweetheart," she says, smiling and stroking a cheek with the back of her index finger. "Ready for some milk and a little cuddle?"

1730: 5:30 P.M.

Time for Board Rounds. All L&D rooms are filled, except for PAR.

In Special Delivery, there's a young woman named Bethany Kidder who has been under a private midwife's care. In advanced labor, she has come to Pill Hill because the midwife wanted assurances that she would be paid for her delivery.

In Room 16, Jessica Dunham is being sent home. Another false alarm, the second in three weeks.

Room 10 contains a woman named Marcia Piatnek.

In Room 8, Rachel Ochs is hoping this is it.

In the Exam Room, Colette Fitzgerald and Kristi Long are both waiting to be examined.

1822: 6:22 P.M.

Dr. E. Paul Kirk, in brown tweed jacket and brown slacks, looking almost extraterrestrial among the green scrubs, talks with Carrie Huston, his private patient.

When she called the hospital, thinking her membranes had ruptured, they insisted she come right in, rather than wait for tomorrow's scheduled appointment with the department chairman.

"I suspect that the leaking you're experiencing is just some leftover urine, rather than ruptured membranes," says the

Englishman. She will probably be sent home, he tells her.

"Honey, you'd better call the airport and see if you can catch Mom," Carrie tells her husband, who stands beside the bed. Her mother's plane is due to land at Portland International in about five minutes.

Dr. Kirk leaves Resident Gary Hoffman to do the examination. As he exits the room, he greets Fili, who is carrying several bottles of Betadine down the hall toward the Special Delivery Room.

1931: 7:31 P.M.

In the coffee/supply room, Gary Hoffman, twirling lukewarm spaghetti, which was ferried up from South Hospital's cafeteria, tells of Dr. Kirk's expression when he got a load of the contents of Special Delivery.

"It was..." He tries. "It was like...oh, I can't really describe it!"

The group—two other residents, a nurse—laughs. They've seen it themselves. In fact, special little errands are being devised to go into Special Delivery to get a peek at the scene.

Shades of the late sixties. Or early seventies, starting with the powerful incense being burned. On the bed lies Bethany Kidder, a beautiful twenty-two-year-old woman with one long mahogany braid, dark and lustrous. Striding around the bed, glaring at anyone who dares approach his woman, is Damien, thin and ponytailed, wearing faded jeans and a once-red T-shirt that says AMADEUS.

"No *intervention!*" he bellows at everyone—to doctor, to nurse, to student, even to Fili, as she enters and leaves the room to replenish supplies.

"No *intervention!*"

Along with the couple are three others. A tall, dark, gaunt, thirtyish woman with waist-length hair says she is "related by spirit" to the couple. One man, who says his name is Pluto, wears a white jacket of quilted gauze, white pants, and big, heavy boots of a strange dark leather. He has a long, scraggly beard and long hair topped with a white safari hat. Around his neck, suspended from a leather thong, is what appears from a short distance to be the severed head of some small, unlucky animal. The third man, wearing blue jeans and a fringed vest evidently fashioned from a South American rug, has, in place of a right hand, a lethal-looking hook.

Through the haze of incense emanate dissonant tones, the music of Ravi Shankar from a tape player on the window ledge.

They are all musicians, Damien announces importantly to the people who come and go in the room. (After he has made sure that the intruder isn't intent upon slipping Bethany a pill, or injecting her with some noxious pain-killer.) They play anything from acid rock to R&B to jazz to classical. And they wanted and planned for a home birth. Counted on it.

"And that midwife! She wanted money up front! *Up front!* And we're on *welfare!*" he rants, indignant.

Well, when Bethany was obviously in labor, and the midwife wouldn't come unless they paid her, they knew they might as well just come on up to the Hill and have the baby for nothing. Not that they want to be here, understand? It's just that they *have* to be here. But don't try any of that intervention stuff, or any of those pain-killers or anything. They know what hospitals are like, and they want the baby naturally.

Understand? Get it? No intervention!

On the bed, Bethany Kidder lies, ignored by all but the nurses and doctors who come in and out to check on the progress of her labor. She wishes it didn't hurt so much. She wishes, in fact, she could have something for the pain. Not to knock her out or anything like that, just something so it wouldn't hurt so much. But how can she ask for it, with Damien being such an asshole?

2107: 9:07 P.M.

In the coffee/supply room, Nurse Susan Cech tells the group, which is eating fudge brownies—still warm!—that she's changing jobs, moving into the clinic to work with the midwives.

"It's been the most *intense* six months of my nursing career," she says. But she's just not an adrenaline junkie.

Nurse-Midwife Carol Howe and Chief Resident Ilona Torok talk about the classical stereotypes, which they say are true, of doctors in different specialties:

Surgeons are arrogant, rude, obnoxious, demanding, and egotistical.

Anesthesiologists aren't too interested in patients as people: The only good patient is an unconscious patient.

Dermatologists like the fact that they rarely lose a patient.

OBs genuinely like people, and don't mind hearing about their patients' personal problems.

2115: 9:15 P.M.

In Room 16, a Polynesian family has been gathered for an hour around Gracie Helu, twenty-five, who moans and shakes with a huge contraction. Gracie's husband, a slender, dark, handsome, and moustached man sporting a white baseball cap saying DALLAS COWBOYS, is intent on the Trail Blazers game on the TV screen at the end of the room. He tells the nurses that they come from Tonga, near Fiji, and that they graduated from the University of Hawaii.

Near the door, the couple's three-year-old son Joel plays with his cousin Tommy, who is four. Every few minutes, Joel moves to the end of the bed to gaze in horrified fascination at his mother's exposed genitalia, his expression not unlike that of a child peering into a bucket of worms.

Tommy's mother—Gracie's sister—tells the little boys to stay quiet. The laboring woman pulls hard on the edges of her husband's navy blue jacket. A lone tear trickles down her left cheek. Eyes fixed on the television screen—the Blazers are up against the Golden State Warriors—Gracie's husband drapes a casual hand over Gracie's head, absently stroking her long, dark hair.

Their son Joel begins to cry, loudly. Cynthia Fairfax, a pretty blond medical student, is holding back Gracie's right leg, and Nurse Carolyn Bachhuber does the same with the left leg as the woman pushes hard.

255

Almost conversationally, Resident Gary Hoffman asks the couple if their three-year-old understands what's about to happen.

"Nah," says Joel's father, glancing down briefly at his son.

"In that case," suggests Dr. Hoffman, "why don't we put him in one place and keep him there? Like in the corner over there behind the bed?"

As the little boy is relocated, Med Student Cynthia puts a blue gown over her green scrubs and dons sterile plastic gloves. Despite the professional regalia, with her golden-red hair caught back in a barrette, she looks more like Alice in Wonderland than a doctor-in-training.

Over by the door, Gracie's nephew Tommy sits on a stool and faces the wall, pretending to drive a car.

"*Vrooom! Vrooom! Vrooom!*" says the four-year-old.

"*Uuuuuh!*" says the laboring woman.

"*Waaahhh!*" cries Joel, ignored and corraled in the corner behind the bed.

The shouting of the basketball crowd on the television sounds tinny, distant.

With one final, heroic push, a baby is born.

"*All right!*" says Dr. Gary Hoffman. "And it's a"—he gently pries small legs apart—"*girl!*"

The father, looking down, grins happily.

"I'm hungry!" says the mother.

"*Vroom! Vroom! Vroom!*" says the four-year-old.

From the corner behind the bed, Joel cries piteously.

"I wanna *go!*" he weeps. "I wanna *go!*"

He crawls out from under the bed and is lured from his mother's side by promises of candy. His cousin Tommy follows.

"I don't speak English," Tommy announces without a trace of accent.

"Ah, I see," says the woman who has removed the children from the delivery room.

"Why is night time?" he asks her in the elevator on the way down to the canteen.

A half hour or so later, the woman is rocking Joel in the chair with broken arms, singing to him in the hall outside

Room 16. He takes his right thumb from his mouth and tells her he doesn't want to go back into that room. She tells him he doesn't have to. The thumb pops back into the three-year-old's mouth.

In the coffee/supply room, Residents Kathleen Doyle and Julie Bouchard talk about a couple Kathy's heard about. He's fifty-eight and she's thirty-two, and they're having their rhinoplasties done the same day. His-and-hers noses.

CHAPTER EIGHTEEN

DAY 11: Thursday, April 21

("I don't know the Cantonese word for 'placenta,' " apologizes the jaunty medical student.)

1533: 3:33 P.M.

A COOL APRIL AFTERNOON, the rain steady outside the windows of the coffee/supply room.

Samantha Ames, a seventeen-year-old private nurse-midwifery patient, has been on L&D since noon, laboring in Room 2. As of ten minutes ago, her baby has been determined to be in significant distress, and the patient is being readied for a crash c-section. No time for an epidural: She has to be given a general anesthetic, knocked out completely.

L&D springs into action. Anesthesiology Resident Amy Ream and Staff Doctor William Owens prepare her in OR2. Chief Resident Nicholas Abrudescu and Residents Tracey Delaplain and Julie Bouchard scrub up in the adjacent room. So does Staff Doctor John Bissonnette, who will oversee the surgery. Nurses Jeanne Gates and Erika Byers are putting on masks and caps, as are Medical Student Lorie Morgan and Nurse-Midwife Tom Lloyd.

In OR2 the young woman's belly is scrubbed with bright orange Betadine and draped, the cover brought up in front of her face to shield her from the sight of the proceedings. Samantha's boyfriend holds her hand as the doctors on the other side of the drape prepare her belly. The patient shudders, making a moaning, terrified sound.

"It's okay, Sam!" the boyfriend says. "It's going to be okay!"

Okay? That's not how anyone would describe what happens next. It is an anesthesiologist's—and a surgeon's—bad dream.

When a patient is being given a general anesthetic, put completely out, there is a crucial period of time involved. The anesthesiologists induce the unconscious state, transporting the patient into a sleep so profound that the body no longer remembers to breathe. *Curare,* harvested from the bark of certain trees in the Amazon jungle—the same poison used on arrow tips by warring natives—is used to paralyze the chest muscles briefly. Thus, the patient can be intubated, have a tube put down her throat so that a breathing machine can start its work.

There is an interval of only fifteen to thirty seconds to put that tube down the patient's throat.

On this particular April afternoon, in the event of this particular pregnant teenager's crash cesarean section, they cannot get the stubborn tube down the throat of Samantha Ames. The staff anesthesiologist and the resident seem to be squabbling about how to do it. They pull the tube back up, and it is bloody. Residents and nurses, looking at one another over their masks of blue-green paper, roll their eyes.

The baby is in danger: He *must be gotten out or he will die!*

Dr. Bissonnette asks for a needle with some lidocaine, to begin locally anesthetizing the patient's belly. The needle he is handed is too fine, S-curving against the taut orange satin that is Samantha Ames's skin. Nurse-Midwife Tom Lloyd hies himself from OR2. He swiftly brings back another, stronger needle from the coffee/supply room.

The anesthesiologists attempt to suction the blood from the patient's throat. The suction machine stops working. Once again, Tom Lloyd leaves the room, quickly fetching a replacement suction machine.

1551: 3:51 P.M.

The patient is now intubated. Anesthesiology tells the operating doctors that she's out.

The scalpel makes the first slice in the young woman's belly.

The patient is not out.

Seventeen-year-old Samantha Ames, tube down her throat, makes a horrible gurgle, an odd high-pitched sound, the scream of a small young animal, mortally wounded.

The surgical team waits another minute or so.

The patient is out, completely unconscious, yes yes yes.

Working fast, the doctors excavate a bellowing little boy, who is swiftly cleaned up and examined, wrapped in warm blankets, and rushed to the INCU.

Samantha Ames's son weighs five pounds twelve ounces. His Apgar score is 9.

He is just fine. His name is Colin Montgomery Ames.

It's okay, the doctors and nurses say among themselves in the coffee/supply room, once it's all over. It's okay, really. She won't remember. If you ask Samantha Ames what's the last thing she remembers, once she's out of it, she'll say she only remembers counting backward. We had to get that kid out. It was a mistake. It happens.

It's *not* okay, says Nicholas Abrudescu, it's not okay at all. It's horrifying. And it's terrible for the baby, that sharp, sudden rush of adrenaline to the mother, going straight into the baby's system.

But nobody's kidding himself or herself. There was nothing okay about what happened this afternoon in OR2. Everybody feels cruddy about it.

1602: 4:02 P.M.

The rubble in Special Delivery has deepened in the nearly twenty-four hours that Bethany Kidder's coterie has been in residence. On the window ledge is a vase of purply roses and a basket of pink and yellow tulips arranged with other spring blooms. The ledge also boasts an empty Thermos bottle, a half dozen discarded milk cartons, three yogurt containers, with custardy smears all over the outside, a teddy bear-shaped plastic honey dispenser, a small electric pot for heating water, and four banana peels, darkening and curling, rotting odoriferously in the warm delivery room.

After resisting getting Pitocin to move her labor along, Bethany finally relented earlier this afternoon. (Over the vociferous objections of her boyfriend, Damien, and their three friends, who urged the laboring young woman to "Hang in there—we know you can do it *naturally*!")

In the room, as Bethany's labor is finally coming to fruition, are the original party, Nurse Doreen Liebertz, a nursing student, and a newcomer. Standing aside, regarding her daughter's friends with transparent distaste, Bethany's mother wears a surplice-styled teal silk blouse and slacks of magenta-hued raw silk.

Ping! goes the air conditioner. *Ping! Ping! Ping!*

Completely nude, her dark-nippled breasts slick with sweat, Bethany leans back against the bed, which is cranked into a sitting position. Damien holds his arm around her shoulders, his thin biceps bulging as she pushes with each contraction.

Tracey Delaplain injects Novocain into Bethany's perineum, and slices the episiotomy as Damien gasps, squeezing his eyes shut and turning his head away.

"I think I'm gonna heave," he says in a gargly voice.

In one swift motion, barely looking his way, a nurse hands Damien a plastic basin he begins retching into.

At last, an eight-pound boy emerges.

"*Skin to skin!*" shouts the father, shoving his barf-filled basin onto the window ledge, next to the tulips and rotting banana peels. "*Skin to skin!*"

The doctors and nurses have become very tired of this man: What, pray tell, is he talking about?

"Give him to her! Let her hold him!" He is wild-eyed, a madman wildly gesticulating.

The new father is assured that this is exactly what they

are planning to do, if they can just cut the cord first. Would he care to do the honors?

Damien cuts his son's umbilical cord.

Pluto, the man in the safari hat, still wearing the animal head on a thong around his neck, is arm in arm with his long-haired girlfriend, and the two of them form a three-way embrace with the new father. The new grandmother, who has remained at a distance throughout, looks at the trio as though upon alien creatures.

After a brief hesitation, Bethany's mother clears her throat.

"What are you going to name him?" she finally asks her daughter.

"How do we know?" snaps Damien before Bethany can speak. "We won't know what his name is until we get to *know* him a little." He shakes his head: Some people are so dumb!

A few minutes later, Nurse Doreen prepares to leave the room and its occupants. Just before opening the door, she turns and speaks.

"*You*," she says to the assembly. "*You* are going to clean up this room before you leave it!"

Once she's safely out of the room, Damien speaks.

"Jeez!" he says to the others. "Can you *believe* this place?"

Without a word, the long-haired woman, she with the man in safari hat and thonged animal head, begins to gather up the rubble. The new grandmother joins her in the task.

Ping! goes the air conditioner. *Ping! Ping! Ping!*

1831: 6:31 P.M.

It's pouring rain outside the windows in the empty coffee supply room. In the hall, Third-Year Medical Student Andrew Yao Tao Su lopes toward the nursing station. Number-one son of a doctor, grandson of a doctor, great-grandson of his family's first doctor, missionary-trained back in China, the twenty-five-year-old with the glasses and perpetual slight smile leans slightly into some unseen wind as he walks, springing lightly on the balls of his feet.

"How's your Chinese, Andy Su?" someone asks.

263

"Depends on the dialect," he replies, gazing at The Board on the wall behind the nurses' station. "I was only ten when we left Hong Kong."

There is a reason for the question. In Room 2 lies Mei Chan, a thirty-seven-year-old Chinese woman who speaks no English. Her husband, who has some English, is with her. "A wonderful couple," the nurses have pronounced them. While Mr. Chan's English is useful for many things, the laboring woman needs to be able to understand what the doctor will tell her as the birth comes closer.

The medical student Andy Su picks up the chart of Mei Chan and studies it so that he will know as much as possible about the patient before he goes into Room 2 to complete her intake.

Even under ordinary circumstances, medical students doing their OB/GYN rotation on 4NE play a very useful part in the workings of the labor and delivery floor. It's a trade-off that works well for everyone. The student is there to learn how to initially "work up" the newly arrived patient—to get a history of the previous medical care, if any, to go over any available medical records, then write up the admission notes. Is she truly in labor? Are her membranes ruptured? Then, the findings are presented to the resident in charge. Often, the student will give the woman a pelvic exam, but in the presence of the more experienced resident. In return for this sort of scutwork, the students are taught how to do uncomplicated deliveries. Depending on the circumstances, students may also "scrub in" on cesarean sections, holding retractors and helping to blot up blood. Between these chores, they spend a lot of time waiting around for patients to come in.

If a patient assigned to a medical student becomes high-risk or complicated, the student's part in her care diminishes. The secretarial, note-taking role will remain, but the student is unlikely to be actively involved in the eventual delivery of the child.

Andy Su suspects that his role in Mei Chan's delivery will be limited to acting as her translator, once he's examined her and asked all the appropriate questions. Nobody else for miles around will know how to find out when she had her last menstrual period, if her pregnancy has been okay, when her contractions began.

Third-Year Medical Student Andrew Yao Tao Su is happy he is on tonight, proud to be of very specific use this rainy April evening on 4NE.

The Board shows that all the other labor rooms are filled, save one.

Debbie Pellegrini is up from MBU and lies in the PAR. But she's pretty clearly not in active labor. Could be the pizza is giving her stomach pains.

In Room 16, Maya Turnquist, twenty-two, was admitted at three this afternoon, and, unlike many of the women on 4NE, is actually in labor at forty weeks, at "normal" term.

Barbara Reingold, in Room 10, has been in the Mother-Baby Unit for four weeks.

Colette Fitzgerald, who came in yesterday and was sent down to MBU, is back up again, this time in Room 8.

Penny Beard, a twenty-year-old, is in the Exam Room being told by Resident Tracey Delaplain that she can go back home.

The word is that the Chinese couple has a three-year-old daughter. If Mei Chan has a son, she is to be scheduled to have her tubes tied tomorrow.

If the baby is another girl, she will not be sterilized.

Andy Su has been more or less planning to become a doctor ever since he can remember. There was no moment of dazzling insight, no *eureka!* It's the family business. Not that his parents put pressure on him. When he was in high school in suburban Lake Oswego, winning all those prizes for his piano talent, he got to thinking about making a career in music. Music is a good career when you're one of the few famous artists. Otherwise, it's really hard to make a steady living. And the lifestyle's very tough, you know, traveling all the time. That didn't appeal much. Being able to play and be creative, that appealed a lot to Andy. Medicine, you're not expected to be creative. You're expected to be objective all the time.

Then, when he was an undergraduate at Stanford, Andy Su discovered political science, found it exciting. Still, his parents told him to go ahead, study what he wanted to. So, he majored in both biology and political science. Maybe he could go for a doctorate in poli-sci and teach at the college level. That would be fine. Or join the foreign service, spend his life living all over the world. An exciting life like that—that would be great! Still, though, there was a family tradition to uphold.

Until the late nineteenth century, the Su family were farmers, living in what is now called Fujian Province in Southern China. Then Yuk Bun Su, who would become Andy Su's great-grandfather, was trained as a doctor by American missionaries, learning his trade in much the same way his twenty-five-year-old great-grandson is presently learning in an American university: by apprenticing, working alongside trained doctors. Yuk Bun Su's wife was a midwife, delivering more than two thousand babies over the many years of her life. That couple's son, Tsan-en Su, who would become Andy Su's grandfather, received a formal education in medicine, studying at St. John's University, a hospital and medical school in Shanghai. He met Andy's grandmother-to-be, a nurse, there. Andy's father, Chung Yee Su, trained to become a doctor at the University of Hong Kong, a British school.

After practicing for many years in Hong Kong, Tsan-en Su, Andy's grandfather, decided to go to America, to Dearborn, Michigan, where two of his sons—one of whom had a doctorate in chemistry, the other a doctorate in physics—had settled. He took and passed the licensing test for foreign medical school graduates, then went to America, where he was eligible to do a residency position. At sixty-two, Tsan-en Su began a three-year internal medicine residency at Oakwood Hospital in Dearborn, emerging to practice medicine for a half dozen years before retiring. He didn't have to keep on practicing, to go through another residency. He just wanted to continue with his part of the family's tradition. At forty, wanting wider educational opportunities for his children, Andy's father, Chung Yee Su, followed his father and brothers, and left a thriving private practice in Hong Kong to begin a family practice residency at Dearborn's Oakwood Hospital.

Andy had little first-hand observation of any occupation other than medicine and health care. His father's sister is an obstetrician/gynecologist. Andy's mother is a physical therapist; his uncle is a doctor. An aunt is a pharmacist. His younger brother is about to study medicine. His sister, studying at Southern Methodist University for a master's degree in music (*somebody* in the family is making use of her musical talent, Andy thinks), is engaged to marry an anesthesiologist, an ABC, American-born Chinese. (They tease this prospective family member, calling him a banana—yellow on the outside, white on the inside!) Medicine is not an easy life, they all tell Andy. But it is a rewarding experience, emotionally. Also it's a steady-type job. You don't worry about a lot of things.

In the end, Andy opted for medical school. It was a relief to be accepted at OHSU, so he wouldn't be such a financial burden to his family. While he was at Stanford, he took out student loans, but his parents paid for the rest of it. Andy's father has returned to Hong Kong to practice medicine. After the first couple of years, when he lived in an apartment near the med school, Andy lives again in the family's home in Lake Oswego. His mother continues to commute back and forth to Hong Kong.

The only time he felt he had no goal was the first few months after he got into medical school. He'd been working toward being right where he was since high school. For six, seven years, his goal was to get into med school, and he felt lost! Now he's set another goal: to become an internist. That's three years of a residency. Then he can subspecialize. Cardiology or gastroenterology, probably.

Being on L&D these past few weeks, helping the babies get born, has been fun. But the lifestyle is tough. And to tell the truth, the way insurance is, it's just not worth it. Even established obstetricians are stopping delivering babies because they can't afford it anymore. People have that thing about the guaranteed perfect baby, and if something—anything—goes wrong, they figure it's the doctor's fault. The hours don't appeal either, but it's exciting. It's *really* exciting.

What he finds he likes a lot is the intellectual aspect of medicine. Internal medicine is like a *puzzle*, intricate and intriguing. Someone comes in really sick, they've seen two or three doctors, but nobody can figure out what's going on. Multiple organ failures, multiple diseases. And you're able to pinpoint all that to *one cause*. It's a lot more like detective work, though the hours aren't a whole lot better than OB.

Andy likes the idea of marrying and having children, but it's going to be a while. He has to be career-oriented now, keep that focus. To be an internist, go someplace and do his residency, and at the end of it, do a fellowship in either cardiology or gastroenterology. Probably, he'll marry along the way, but he doesn't think it would be fair to have children until he's established himself.

His parents, though, they urge him to marry soon, to start a family. They tease him about it. When you get through with all your work and you're established, you'll be an old man! And if you have a little baby, by the time the baby grows up, you'll be an old, old man!

It will probably be better to marry a girl who's Asian, preferably one with a Chinese background. That will be easier for him, easier for his family. Not that it matters that much to Andy himself. His family is still very Chinese in a lot of ways. They're a close family, and when they get together, Andy's mom prepares stuff and they all eat with chopsticks.

It's more than just food, though. Asian parents, when they come into the hospital to have a baby, usually say, especially if they already have other children, "If male, tubal ligation." He doesn't know how many times the nurses and residents and others have noticed that. It happens a *lot* with Asians, especially Chinese. They have this thing about having boys in the family. It's on the chart of Mei Chan, who is in labor in Room 2. Mei Chan will try again—and again and again, if necessary—until her family is "completed" by the birth of a son.

That's typically Chinese, a custom, an old world type of thing. When the white patients say they want a tubal ligation, Andy will ask, "Regardless of sex?" and they just look at him funny. Even though they might have two or three boys already, or two or three girls.

Another thing different about being Chinese is the way you interact with elders. You're supposed to be more respectful, a little bit more reverent. Here, individual expression, freedom of ideas, and just being articulate, able to tell people how you feel, is respected, regarded as a very positive thing. Over in the old world, in China, it's not like that.

Custom. Tradition. That's why Andy thinks his parents would prefer him to marry a Chinese girl. He can understand their feeling. But if the right person comes along, and he fell in love, he *knows* his parents would adjust. They all understand one another very well. They trust him. They let him go to college away from home, didn't make any hassles. They supported him through his education. Basically, they were there whenever he needed them. And when he needed to go, they would let him go. So he couldn't ask anything more of them.

1952: 7:52 P.M.

Bethany Kidder, down in the Mother-Baby Unit, tells her boyfriend she's definitely glad she had her still-unnamed son in the hospital. Damien, scowling and sprawled in the chair alongside her bed, is angry. He's mad that after his son was born, they didn't let them all just stay in the room and *glow in it.* Now he's just learned that before they can take their son home, the infant must have a drug screen. As if Bethany did drugs. Pot doesn't count, not really.

And he's still pissed at that stupid midwife wanting money from them.

Hilary Blanchard puts down her needlepoint and glances at the front-page headlines of *The New York Times.* Nothing there to get too excited about. She turns to the crossword. One across: *Starry.* Hmmmm...Seven across: *N.H. city....* Thirteen across: *Qualm....* Fifteen across: *Skeptically....* Seventeen across: *Place for a cradle?* Eighteen across: *Small pianos.* SPINETS!

Richie is taking her mother out to dinner tonight. Hilary told them to go to Jake's Famous Crawfish. And to bring her back a nice big piece of that chocolate truffle cake.

1932: 7:52 P.M.

Harriet Grackle, waiting to be examined, her husband, Animal, sitting beside her holding her hand, remembers

269

something she read somewhere. Maybe from a book her four-year-old son Tommy was given.

"Isn't there something about how a mother elephant is pregnant two years? Is that it?" Harriet squirms her swollen body around to look at Animal.

"Baby, you do not look like an elephant," says her mate. "If that's what you're trying to say." A kind man, this biker, a true gentleman who in the past difficult month has assured his wife that she doesn't look puffy, not a bit. Truth to tell, these days Harriet Grackle bears some resemblance to the Pillsbury Doughboy. Indeed, Animal Grackle looks forward to welcoming his baby, and to seeing his onetime-dancer wife regain her mind-boggling figure.

Harriet knows you're not supposed to drink when you're pregnant. But by God, tonight she had a beer. Then she had a funny feeling about an hour ago, and maybe that's labor?

"Animal, what do you think chances are of getting them to induce labor for me tonight?" she asks.

"Slim to none, babe," he answers. "Slim to none." Shifting his hulk in the itsy-bitsy chair beside the exam table holding Harriet, he leans his head forward to kiss his wife's puffy hand.

A resident enters the room, asks a few questions, palpates Harriet Grackle's enormous belly, and sends the couple on their way.

"You know how to get back out of here?" asks the resident.

"Why yes, I believe we do!" says Animal Grackle, right elbow angled out for his wife to take for support.

Down the hall. Into the elevator. Out to the parking lot. Helmets on. Onto the elderly Harley Panhead. And back through the driving rain, to a small house in St. Johns in North Portland.

2032: 8:32 P.M.

Medical Student Andy Su, born in Hong Kong and soon to be the fourth generation of doctors in his family, is coaching Mei Chan in her native dialect. Everyone is pleased by the happy coincidence that Andy can speak Cantonese, one of dozens of Chinese dialects. And it is further coincidental that he happens to be on this shift, on this rotation, tonight.

Resident Tracey Delaplain, feeling especially pregnant herself, crouches forward from a stool at the end of the bed, checking on the laboring woman's progress.

"I'm sure glad you're here," she tells the medical student. "How old were you when you left Hong Kong?"

"Ten," replies Andy. "And there are certain words I don't know." He searches his mind for the Cantonese word for placenta. No luck.

"Okay," says Dr. Delaplain. "Here comes a contraction. Tell her to push."

"*Tuai! Tuai!*" Push! Push!

Mei Chan, smooth golden skin gleaming with perspiration, bears down and pushes with all her strength. Her husband, a small and tidy man, holds an arm under his wife's head. He is clad in freshly pressed tan chinos and a pink shortsleeved shirt with green and white cross-hatching.

"*Dai leg dee!*" urges Andrew Yao Tao Su. Harder!

Mei Chan's husband wipes her gleaming face with a wet washcloth and makes grunting sounds along with her as she works. The contraction ends.

"*Fong-sung,*" says the medical student. Relax.

Mei Chan's husband puts his face up to hers, murmuring softly and rubbing his nose on her forehead.

The fetal heart monitor shows another contraction beginning.

"Tell her to push *real hard* this time," Resident Tracey Delaplain instructs Andy Su.

"*Tuai, tuai,*" he says, rocking from one leg to the other. "*Tuai, tuai—dai leg dee!*"

Mei Chan's husband, standing beside her head, holds both her hands and squeezes them.

The episiotomy, and then the baby.

It is a boy.

The father sobs and kisses his wife on the mouth. She has tears running down her cheeks.

"*Doh tsei ley, yau yat kor tsai ah!*" says the husband of Mei Chan, over and over. "*Doh tsei ley, yau yat kor tsai ah! Doh tsei ley, yau yat kor tsai ah!*"

Only Andrew Yao Tao Su, number-one son, soon to be

the fourth-generation doctor of his family, knows what is being said is this:

"Thank you, my wife, for my son."

2225: 10:25 P.M.

Every labor room is empty except for Room 16, where Maya Turnquist feels an occasional contraction and watches a sexy woman judge hire *L.A. Law*'s sleazoid Arnold Becker to represent her in a divorce case.

In the INCU, crack cocaine addict Timothy Edwards, who has learned to suck really well, is being rocked and given a bottle by the nurse named Mary.

The nurses in L&D—Doreen Liebertz, Patti Spooner, and Natasha McLeron—jacked up by too much coffee and excitement earlier in the afternoon, are making work for themselves. Doreen (who swore she wasn't going to end up doing it) is wiping down the windowsill in Special Delivery, scraping off the last of the gummy yogurt with her right thumbnail. She is shaking her head, muttering something under her breath. Over near the bed, Fili Cox is mopping the floor.

In Room 8, Resident Tracey Delaplain sits in a chair, feet elevated (as she often advises other pregnant women to do), hands folded across her rounded belly, as she watches *Heartbeat*. She wishes aloud that someone would do a TV series about doctors and hospitals that tells it like it really *is*.

At the end of the hall by the operating rooms, Charge Nurse Denise Reed is neatening up a pile of papers.

In the coffee/supply room, Resident Jan Leigh holds out her left hand in front of her, in customary gesture as she shows off her new wedding ring to Julie Bouchard.

Down in the Mother-Baby Unit, Mei Chan sits up in bed, her husband sitting in the chair beside her, smiling, smiling, smiling. Their three-year-old daughter sits cross-legged at the foot of the bed. The three of them talk rapidly—in Cantonese—while feasting upon takeout containers of Kung Pao Chicken with chopsticks.

In the bassinet next to the bed, a small son sleeps, one long journey ended, and another just begun.

The moment of quiet on 4NE won't last for long.

In Northwest Portland's Willamette Heights, a thirty-nine-year-old lawyer, a primipara named Elinor Bollinger, lies with her husband in their bed, a mahogany four-poster handed down through her family for over two hundred years. She has, in fact, spent most of the past three months in this bed, holding on to her in vitro fertilized pregnancy with its three babies within.

Whoosh! Elinor Bollinger feels a wetness between her legs. Amniotic fluid soaks through Elinor's flannel nightgown, through the ironed cotton sheets, through the mattress pad, making a stain she will smile at in the years to come.

Her labor has begun.

"Ted," she says softly. "Ted? Wake up, honey. My time's come. Let's get going up that hill."

Across the Willamette River, in Northeast Portland, a fifteen-year-old black girl named KaLishia Garfield watches a movie on television, sitting cross-legged on the floor of the living room.

Whoosh! KaLishia Garfield feels like she's peeing, a wild gush of warm fluid coming out all over her legs, all over the worn pattern of the linoleum. KaLishia knows what it is, since this will be her second baby with Ron.

Her labor has begun.

"Mama?" she calls into the kitchen. "Mama? Is La-Shaunda's car fixed yet? My time's come. We better get up that hill."

At the foot of Marquam Hill, a rambling, drafty Victorian house on Southwest Corbett contains three couples dwelling communally, the men all members of a heavy-metal rock group called Void Where Prohibited. Tonight, they're playing at a murky downtown tavern called Satyricon, sharing the bill with Sweaty Nipples, Smegma, and Vomit Lunch. At the kitchen sink stands a twenty-two-year-old named Bettina Shemansky, her cropped hair moussed into lethal-looking spikes of Day-Glo pink, green, and orange. Her huge belly keeps her almost a foot away from the single sink where she's finally washing up three days' worth of food-encrusted, unmatching dishes. It's not her turn to do this, and she is not pleased. Not pleased at all.

Whoosh! Bettina Shemansky feels a gush of warm fluid. It splashes onto the ugly green indoor-outdoor carpet. Someone else can clean it up.

Her labor has begun.

"Serena!" she calls from the kitchen. "Serena! Desdemona! My time's come. Let's get our ass up that fucking hill!"

And so it goes. Coming up Pill Hill from all over the city, the women will make their way to 4NE, one after another, night after night, some 250 each month. Mostly, they will be unable to pay. And mostly, everything will turn out all right.

Elinor Bollinger, whose pregnancy is only six months old, will labor for eight hours, and end up being delivered by cesarean section. After a month in the Intermediate Neonatal Care Unit, her triplet sons will all do well. After briefly considering dubbing them Curly, Moe, and Larry, the Bollingers will name their hard-won progeny Geoffrey, Michael, and Thomas.

KaLishia Garfield, whose sister LaShaunda's car was not fixed, will finally arrive at 4NE by ambulance. Fifteen minutes after she is tucked into the Special Delivery Room at the end of the hall, she will be delivered of a daughter. When her boyfriend, Ron, arrives, around midnight, the little girl will be named Ronyetta.

Bettina Shemansky, who has been coming faithfully to the outpatient clinic for her checkups, will have a nine-pound son.

Her boyfriend, christened Brian but now glorying in the name Siegfried and wearing his hair in a Mohawk, will make it from Satyricon in time to cut the umbilical cord of his firstborn, whom he will want to name Elvis.

He will settle for Dominick.

EPILOGUE

And Then What Happened to Them All

When I passed through the swinging doors at the end of 4NE's hallway for the last time late one April night in 1988, I knew I was going to miss it all. An adrenaline junkie myself, I knew that withdrawing from life on the Labor and Delivery Department at Oregon Health Sciences University was going to be tough. I knew I'd miss the thrill of being in the room while a labor builds to its crescendo, feeling my heart thumping wildly as a child emerged. I wanted to continue to bear witness to the appearance of one more beautiful, astounding little human being.

I knew I was going to miss them, all of them. Staff doctors and residents, nurses and midwives, patients and their new babies and their families. I'd come to care—a lot, in some cases—for the people whose paths crossed mine during my adventures on 4NE, there atop Portland's Marquam Hill. Again and again, engrossed in each tale of sadness and triumph, I was struck by how courageous people can be, how sometimes carrying on is the most a person can do. I knew I'd miss the cookies and coffee, holding hands during labors, sitting in hallways and in the cafeteria. I'd miss listening and taking notes, filling dozens of tiny tapes. Yet, when I drove down off Pill Hill that last night to start writing their stories, they all became fixed in time for me. In order to get them down right, I had to freeze-frame them all. Forever pregnant. Forever trying to get pregnant. Forever lashed to drug addictions or to being on welfare or to trying to get through one more sleepless night of residency.

Ah, but life does goes on. From time to time, I'd hear about the changes among "my" residents and "my" patients. Finally, nearing completion of my book, I tracked them down to find out where their lives had taken them. Some of what I found out surprised me, and some of it didn't.

First-Year Resident Gary Hoffman—"Darling Doctor Hoffman"—and his wife Ericka, whose firstborn, Alexandra, was a victim of Sudden Infant Death Syndrome, became the parents of a healthy baby boy, Zachary, in May of 1989. Daughter Cassandra continues to do well. At the conclusion of his residency in the summer of 1991, Gary began working for the West Hills Clinic, joining former fellow resident Tim Stewart in a private, six-doctor OB/GYN practice based at Southwest Portland's St. Vincent Hospital.

Nurse-Midwife Nancy Sullivan, who delivered the triploid baby of patient **Julie O'Brien,** left OHSU in May 1990 to become director of clinical services for Healthy Start, a nonprofit corporation providing maternity care to indigent women in nearby Washington County. With a staff of twelve, Healthy Start offers principal care by its half-dozen nurse-midwives. Hispanic women comprise about one half of its clientele. Healthy Start operates out of a modest one-story building shared with a Head Start program for the children of migrant workers, as well as a Hispanic drug and alcohol program.

In many ways a model program of its sort, Healthy Start delivers some forty-five babies each month, and plans are being made to expand its approach to an additional two such clinics in the Portland area. Citing "wonderful support from the local medical community" in Hillsboro, Nancy says she loves working where she is now.

Third-Year Resident Julie Bouchard is the medical director for Healthy Start. She also operates a general private

OB/GYN practice in Aloha, a small town outside Portland. Her months of trying to conceive a child through the rigors of residency paid off: Chelsea Nicole Bouchard Beyerman was born February 3, 1989. (According to the couple's calculations, conception did indeed take place in a residents' call room!) Trained as an environmental engineer, Julie's husband, Glenn, stays home now with Chelsea. The couple has been trying for another child, and Julie has experienced three miscarriages since Chelsea's birth.

First-Year Resident Tracey Delaplain ended up having her baby at OHSU, after all. Patrick Thomas Delaplain was born July 15, 1988. Her parents moved to Portland from Nevada to care for their grandson during the day while Tracey and Tom worked. When Tracey finally finished her residency in the summer of 1991, she moved with her family back to Elko, Nevada, where she joined a private practice.

Giving up on all the elaborate fertility procedures, **Nurse Jeanne Gates** and her husband, Paul, finally achieved parenthood "the normal way." Their son Nicholas Matthew was born on 4NE on April 17, 1989. Less than two years later, on January 11, 1991, Samuel Charles was born. Paul Gates has changed jobs—twice—and works now for a winery in nearby Forest Grove. Jeanne continues a heavy part-time (80 percent) schedule on the three-to-eleven P.M. shift on Pill Hill's L&D.

At the moment Jeanne Gates was giving birth in January of 1991 to her second son, **Charge Nurse Denise Reed** was having her own difficult labor in the adjacent room on the fourth floor of North Hospital atop Marquam Hill. Griffin Kestrel Reed's arrival brought great joy to his parents, who had undergone Denise's miscarriage nearly three years earlier. After that pregnancy, unable to conceive again, she shed fifty pounds on a liquid diet, and immediately became pregnant.

Denise's husband, **Andy,** was accepted into medical school on The Hill, and began his studies in the fall of 1991. Denise, who'd cut back to a half-time schedule after her son's birth, reduced her working hours still more, to 20 percent, accommodating the changes in her family's life brought about by Andy's medical training.

Chief Resident Jan Leigh is now a member of a four-woman private OB/GYN practice based in Northwest Portland's Good Samaritan Hospital. Her husband, **Marc**, continues with his successful woodworking business, and the couple's two children helped celebrate their third anniversary: Katie, born March 30, 1989, and Paul, born March 13, 1991.

Chief Resident Nicholas Abrudescu is in private OB/GYN practice with two other doctors in Worcester, Massachusetts. A year or so after the action of this book, he married a surgical nurse from Pill Hill; the couple has since divorced. No harm came to his family during the political upheaval surrounding the overthrow of Romania's President Ceaucescu. He sees his brother, Florentin, who is completing a residency in New York City, "pretty often."

At the conclusion of her residency, **Chief Resident Elizabeth Newhall** was hired as a member of OHSU's OB/GYN Department. After two years with the department, she joined former fellow resident Jan Leigh in the small private practice at Good Samaritan Hospital. In the summer of 1992, with two other women doctors, Liz plans to open a small clinic, catering to a combination of indigent and paying clients, on Portland's Southeast Hawthorne Boulevard.

Medical Student Andrew Yao Tao Su, the fourth-generation doctor in his family, is well on his way to reaching his professional goal: In June 1992, he will be a chief resident in internal medicine at Oregon Health Sciences University. In April 1990, through a family connection, he began corresponding with Ruby Tan, a graduate student working on a master's degree in statistics in Ohio. Eight months later, they met in person. In June 1991, Andrew Yao Tao Su and Ruby Tan were married in Portland's St. Patrick's Cathedral. They plan to start a family—"maybe next year."

SAFE, an outpatient treatment program for substance-abusing pregnant women, was started on The Hill in November of 1988. As of August 1991, less than three years later, one hundred women had participated in SAFE—an acronym meaning "Substance Abuse Family Evaluation." The program offers substance-abuse counseling, obstetrical care, prenatal education, and child care during the parenting education of its participants. A pediatric physical therapist also works with the babies and their mothers.

Directed by OHSU's Chief of Obstetrics, **Dr. Richard Lowensohn,** SAFE is a joint effort of the university's OB/GYN and psychiatry departments, and also involves the Department of Pediatrics. SAFE was launched with zero funding, then began receiving a small subsidy from the March of Dimes. In January of 1991, the program was awarded a state contract supplying one-half of its operating expenses. Most of SAFE's materials and services, however, continue to be donated.

For all its humble beginnings, SAFE has proven remarkably effective. Roughly 50 percent of the one hundred women enrolled since the program's start went completely off drugs during their pregnancies and 25 percent used significantly less; the other 25 percent didn't do so well.

The Special Delivery Room has been demolished and turned into two labor and delivery rooms, and another L&D room was added on the other side of the swinging doors, bringing the total number of L&D rooms from eight to ten.

To her great relief, after weeks holed up in her private room on Pill Hill's Mother-Baby Unit, **Hilary Blanchard** was allowed to continue her bed rest away from the hospital, as long as she remained in Portland. Staying at the home of friends in Portland Heights, Hilary was able to maintain her in vitro pregnancy, complicated by her incompetent cervix caused by her own mother's use of fertility drugs. In July, about a month premature, it was deemed safe to deliver Hilary's child, a robustly healthy son.

A year or so later, Hilary finally completed the needlework tapestry of "The Unicorn in Captivity." Stretched and framed, it now hangs in the bedroom of Aaron Mitchell Blanchard.

Julie O'Brien, whose triploid baby delivered by Nurse-Midwife Nancy Sullivan died within minutes of delivery, moved with her young son to the East Coast. Living with her mother and stepfather, Julie worked toward restoring order to her life, and to ease her break-up with **Maurice,** father of her dead baby. But Maurice continued courting Julie by telephone, eventually sending an engagement ring.

After six months, Julie returned to Portland to plan a wedding—only to find that, contrary to what she'd been assured, Maurice had been seeing "a string of other women" in her absence. After breaking up another "two or three times," it took another year, she says, to be finally done with him. She has since had "significant relationships" with two other men, though she's seeing nobody now.

Son **Joshua** lives now with his father, who has split with his new wife and moved back to Portland. Julie sees Joshua on alternate weekends, and during school vacations. Julie is working in sales, and continues to find great strength in her friends, and through her church.

Lily Pratt, the extremely obese woman whose risky pregnancy resulted in a normal vaginal delivery of a small son, still lives on the Southern Oregon coast. Since the Pratts have no phone, I drove from Portland to visit. We sat, Lily and I, in the family's cheerfully cluttered living room with its teapot collection and a wall full of souvenir plates while **Scotty Pratt,** now a cheery three-year-old with a thick mop of blond hair, drew a picture for me.

For a long time, Lily told me, the only employment **David Pratt** could find was $5.25-an-hour work as a store security guard. Happily, he recently began working as a railroad safety inspector, earning nearly three times that amount.

Lily stays at home to care for Scotty and her household. She has not lost the weight she hoped to; in fact, she has gained back what was lost on her special pregnancy diet for gestational diabetes. For a while she belonged to Overeaters Anonymous, she says, and it helped show her she isn't alone in her obesity. Now, Lily's doctor has her on a special diabetic diet, and her weight has at least leveled, and seems, she says, to be going down a bit.

Cammie Edwards, the crack-cocaine-addicted young redhead whose son was born in the ambulance, reports that she is off drugs, married to a government worker, and living now in a small town outside Portland with her new husband, his three daughters, and their baby son.

After she broke up with her boyfriend, father of her first three children, Cammie says she stopped using crack, but continued to sell it. She was arrested, convicted as a repeat offender, and recently completed a six-month sentence in the state women's prison in Salem. Arrested with her for peddling crack cocaine, as a first-time offender Cammie's new husband didn't serve any time; he was able to care for the couple's infant son, born while Cammie was still in prison.

Timothy Edwards, born crack-addicted in an ambulance, has remained in the legal custody of his maternal grandmother since birth. Except for "hyper behavior," the red-haired, blue-eyed three-year-old has no lasting results of his cocaine addiction—according to Cammie. Since her release from prison, Cammie sees her three older children regularly, sharing their care with her mother. Within a year, she hopes to have all her children living with her in the newly configured family.

Melody Richards, the eighteen-year-old whose newborn son was adopted by the Mormon couple from Utah, is still adrift, her sister told me. About a year after the arrival of her firstborn, Melody bore a second son, whom she kept. Twenty-one now, still on welfare, Melody is pregnant with her third child. Melody's sister, on learning of this latest pregnancy, urged her not to have an abortion; the new child will probably also be placed for adoption.

Tammy Williams, the eighteen-year-old whose HELLP syndrome—a dangerous variation of pregnancy-induced hypertension—threatened both her life and that of her unborn child, lives now in California, and reported over the phone that she is "very, very happy." Eight months after giving birth to her daughter on 4NE, she married a U.S. Army helicopter pilot. The family, who lives on an army base, now includes a son, born early in 1990.

Zanna Morrison, the twenty-year-old whose cesarean-section delivery was featured in the chapter called "Blood!", married her boyfriend, **Shawn,** when their son was a month old. Zanna went on to take some courses in early childhood education at a local community college, and has done some teaching of preschoolers. Shawn works now as a machinist, and the couple had a second child, a girl, in July of 1991, a month before they moved into a house they bought. Their son has curly blond hair and has recently signed up to model with a local agency; his parents want to start putting money aside for his college education.

One hot August afternoon, I went to visit the patient I call **Debbie Pellegrini.** Debbie—the stroke victim holed up in

283

the Mother-Baby Unit—lives now in a group home for hand-icapped people, sharing (with considerable assistance) a pleasant apartment. While her mind remains as sharp as ever, Debbie still cannot do much for herself, and couldn't care for her baby, born during the summer of 1988.

After the birth of her daughter, Debbie and the child were placed, together, in a foster home. But it didn't work out, and Debbie's mother, who lives in a neighboring state, assumed care of the child. Once in a while, her daughter is brought to Debbie in the group home. Unable to speak, Debbie wrote about it, with great effort, onto my legal pad.

"I had her for one month with me," Debbie wrote. "Then we got separated and I almost lost it." When I looked confused, she added a single word: "Mentally." She continued writing out her story.

"My mom said they were going to adopt her. I wouldn't let her. That is why it hurts."

Unable to be with her little daughter, unable, because of her disability, even to speak of her, Debbie wept as one of her caregivers comforted her from one side, and I from the other.

I told Debbie Pellegrini that I think her little girl is lucky to have her for a mother. That she is very smart, and has a wonderful sense of humor, and that she has a good heart. These things, I told her, are passed along to our children, even when we don't get to be with them.

Then I asked Debbie if she remembered Dr. Gary Hoffman—"DDH." She cheered up, laughed, and clutched her heart in a mock swoon. I promised I'd try to get her a picture of him. Then we opened the tin of homemade cookies I'd brought along.

After weeks of fruitless motorcycle journeys from North Portland to the top of Pill Hill, **Harriet and Animal Grackle** finally had their baby. Happily for all, when Harriet's water finally broke in the middle of the night, **Dr. Gary Hoffman** was in the middle of one of his thirty-six-hour shifts. Harriet had four hours of hard labor, without benefit of Pitocin, and Dr. Hoffman was delighted to deliver what he assured Harriet and Animal was "a good baby," an eight-pound son they named **Herman Leroy Grackle, Jr.** Now three years old, he is called "**Little Animal.**"

With what's come to be called "The Oregon Plan," beginning in July 1992, Oregon's doctors may begin a new relationship with the state's poor patients, in what represents nothing less than a turning point in medical care for America's indigent.

To implement the Oregon Health Plan, the Legislature created an eleven-member Health Services Commission to rank health care services according to their importance. Among the commission's five physicians was **Dr. E. Paul Kirk,** chairman of the department of Obstetrics and Gynecology of Oregon Health Sciences University.

Critics call it "rationing" health care. Supporters call it "prioritizing" care. Proposing nothing less than a dramatic revision of Medicaid, the plan would provide a "Standard Benefit Package" covering every one of the state's citizens whose income falls below the federal poverty line. The tradeoff is that coverage would be denied on certain treatments. "If the physician and patient feel that an uncovered service is vital," Dr. Kirk has said, "care will be provided as it is now—as a charity case."

After countering considerable resistance to the concept of care-by-priority, the plan was made possible by a June 30, 1991, vote by the Oregon legislature providing an additional $33 million to the Medicaid funding already in place.

What's left is for the federal government—the Health Care Financing Administration—to grant a waiver allowing changes in Medicaid coverage. And there is hope for a stamp of approval from Congress. Some Washington opponents think it wrong to deny coverage on certain procedures; others may regard it as a threat to the establishment of national health insurance. In reality, says Dr. Kirk, medical care was already being effectively rationed through Medicaid eligibility rules applying to whole blocks of poor people: men who aren't single parents and women who are neither pregnant nor single parents. While, technically, the congressional waiver is not needed, Oregon wants the support of Congress.

Across the country, and the world, health care professionals and providers are watching the Oregon Health Plan's progress with interest. If everything falls in place, the federal waiver obtained, and the plan indeed implemented in 1992, chances are good that other states will follow suit. If not, Dr. Kirk will, he says, view it as "a striking paradox that while the federal government lays more and more responsibility on the states, it won't allow them to be innovative."

ACKNOWLEDGMENTS

For their generous cooperation, I must express my deep appreciation to the staff of the Labor and Delivery Department of Oregon Health Sciences University. With trust that was immediate and astonishing, they opened up their hearts to me, sharing their work lives and telling their life stories straight into my tape recorder.

The reason for all this trust, of course, is an amazing man named Dr. E. Paul Kirk, Chairman of OHSU's Obstetrics and Gynecology Department. Battling fiscal and bureaucratic odds that would daunt a lesser soul, Dr. Kirk inspires the doctors, nurses, nurse-midwives, and other staff who work with him. His philosophy (indeed, his firm resolve) that all pregnant women deserve to be treated with dignity, that all their babies deserve a good start, is one that inevitably ripples out, powerfully affecting the lives of thousands of women and their families.

Dr. Brian Clark, a resident at the time of the book's action, and later an OB/GYN fellow, deserves a special measure of gratitude. Going over technical details again and again, he generously advised me on baroque medical matters, enriching my understanding—and helping me translate complex medical argot into readable English. I remain grovelingly grateful.

287

Dr. Richard Lowensohn, OHSU Chief of Obstetrics, was most helpful to me, as were Dr. Mark Nichols, head of Pill Hill's OB/GYN residency program, and Nurse-Midwives Nancy Sullivan and Tom Lloyd.

My sincere thanks go to the dozens of patients and their families, who in the midst of intense personal drama (and often pain) were generous in sharing their stories for this book.

Liza Dawson, my editor at Morrow, has guided this book through a number of permutations. I thank her for her patience with this first-time author, as well as for her understanding through the inevitable rough patches. Thanks also to Morrow's Wendy Bellerman for all her help.

Mark Christensen, a gentle and kindly nag—and himself a terrific writer—deserves huge thanks for his encouragement over our years of friendship, and for connecting me with agent provocateur Richard Pine.

My agent Richard Pine has been wonderful from the very start, when I approached him with quite a different book idea. Richard has believed in me, cajoled and cheered me on, and I thank him so much. In Richard's office, Lori Andiman, smart and cheerful, kind and funny, has been marvelous. Every writer should have such terrific people in her corner.

And then there's Katherine Dunn. Brewing endless cups of tea, this brilliant writer has slogged through draft after draft, redefining the word *friendship*. Dr. John Schneider and Barbara Buckingham-Hayes, for reasons well known to them, have been invaluable, and I thank them. Thanks, too, are due The Eastie Boys. The coffee room at Powell's Bookstore has proven to be a good "clean, well-lighted place" in which to work and brood (especially once the snack bar at J. J. Newberry's was shut down); thanks to Anne Hughes for both her friendship and Hellcows.

Special thinks go to my daughters, Jessica Wolk-Stanley and Katherine Wolk-Stanley. They have nurtured, loved, and believed in me when it mattered most. Katy also transcribed countless hours of tapes interviews with 4NE's patients and staff, for which I thank her.

Finally, I thank Samuel Israel Hochberg for his love, support, and constant infusions of Oriental food through the inscrutable process of book writing.

295